S0-BFC-468

How to Write
and Publish
Articles in Nursing

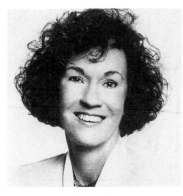

Donna Richards Sheridan, RN, MS, MBA, PhD, is Vice-President of Patient Care/Chief Nurse Executive at Saint Francis Memorial Hospital in San Francisco, California. She has worked as Management Development Coordinator at Stanford University Hospital in Palo Alto, California and was Editor-in-Chief of *Stanford Nurse.* In addition, she is an Associate Professor at the University of California, San Francisco and is on the faculty of the University of Phoenix. She consults and speaks on management development, organizational development, and writing. She is author of *The New Nurse Manager: A Guide to Management Development* (with Bronstein & Walker, 1984) and has four management workbooks published by the National League for Nurses.

She is editor of Mosby's bimonthly *Staff Development Insider,* on the editorial boards of *Journal of Continuing Education in Nursing* and *Nurse Author and Editor.* She has served as editorial consultant to *RN* magazine and was on the Editorial Board of *Health Care Supervisor.* She writes a monthly column as a Board Member of *Aspen's Advisor for Nurse Executives.* She received an award from the American Association of University Women, California State Division, for Outstanding Presidents' Columns.

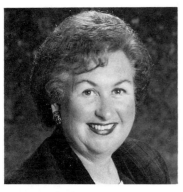

Donna Lee Dowdney, PhD, owns Writing Enterprises International in Palo Alto, California. She consults and presents workshops on writing for publication in healthcare and industry settings and writes and edits books, articles, manuals, and other professional documents.

In addition, she is Chair of the Technical Communications Department and Director of the Student Publications and Design Center at De Anza College. She has delivered presentations at numerous professional conferences. Her professional associations include the American Medical Writers Association, Council of Biology Editors, Society for Technical Communication, and California Writers Club. In 1994 the Society for Technical Communication awarded her the "Distinguished Service Chapter Award" for her work with the Silicon Valley Chapter. In 1996 the Society for Technical Communication awarded her the "President's Award" for her years of dedication to cultivating new technical communicators.

How to Write and Publish Articles in Nursing

Second Edition

Donna Richards Sheridan, RN, MS, MBA, PhD
Donna Lee Dowdney, PhD

 Springer Publishing Company

Copyright © 1997 by Springer Publishing Company, Inc.

All rights reserved

No part of this publication may be reproduced, stored in a
retrieval system, or transmitted in any form or by any means,
electronic, mechanical, photocopying, recording, or otherwise,
without the prior permission of Springer Publishing Company, Inc.

Springer Publishing Company, Inc.
536 Broadway
New York, NY 10012-3955

Cover design by: Margaret Dunin
Production Editor: Pamela Lankas

   98 99 00 01/5 4 3 2

Library of Congress Cataloging-in-Publication Data

Sheridan, Donna Richards.
   How to write and publish articles in nursing / Donna Richards
Sheridan, Donna Lee Dowdney.—2nd ed.
      p.   cm.
   Includes bibliographical references and index.
   1. Nursing—Authorship.   2. Nursing literature—Marketing.
I. Dowdney, Donna Lee.   II. Title.
   [DNLM: 1. Writing—nurses' instruction.   2. Publishing—nurses'
instruction.   WZ 345 S552h   1997]
RT24.S54   1997
0-8261-4981-2
808'.06661—dc21
DNLM/DLC
for Library of Congress   96-49183
                                                                   CIP

Printed in the United States of America

To nurse writers

and

To my husband, Jim,
and my four daughters
Barbra Lyn
Nicole Jenean
Lauren Rebecca
Rachel Anne
and to my parents
William & Lillian Richards

To my husband, Bill,
my daughter, Deborah Lee,
and my son, David Scott

DONNA RICHARDS SHERIDAN

DONNA LEE DOWDNEY

Special thanks to Maryann Zaremska, MLS.

Continuing education credits may be obtained for using this book. For information, contact Donna Richards Sheridan, RN, PhD, 1732 Middlefield Road, Palo Alto, California 94301.

Contents

Foreword: A Nurse Editor's Perspective

Editing and authoring have different and often opposite perspectives. The editor's perspective is naturally, by the scope of the job, a more negative one: looking for problems in a manuscript that can be corrected by editing or rejection and revision. You will notice that editors frequently describe reasons for rejection ("not written to the target audience") and things to avoid ("don't use passive voice").

Meanwhile, the author focuses more on the positive aspects related to writing the manuscript. The successful author focuses more on "what I should do" than on "what I should avoid." There is an important difference in this perspective. If the author dwells on the negative points to avoid, the creativity necessary for writing is reduced, and the positive energy and enthusiasm necessary for avoiding writer's block is abandoned.

In *How to Write and Publish Articles in Nursing*, Donna Richards Sheridan and Donna Lee Dowdney have interviewed numerous successful nursing authors and editors to bring both perspectives to you. The most difficult perspective to present is the author's, yet this book does this very successfully. It is much easier to list what not to do in writing than what to do. Think of your own English classes; you will find that most of the rules describe things not to do, like "do not split infinitives." Here the authors have specific suggestions on what action to take to develop a high-quality manuscript.

From an editor's perspective, the uniqueness of this book is the focus on the writing *process* rather than on rules or reasons for rejection as in other books on writing. Why, from the editor's perspective, is this focus on authoring critical? Because editors know how to edit; they need you to write. Editors have little difficulty editing; we have great difficulty getting good material to edit. The nursing editor's job depends on you, the nurse author; it cannot be done without you.

The nursing journal editor's main responsibility is to develop the journal. This includes:

- targeting the market (deciding what nursing specialties or subspecialties are included in the audience the journal will reach)
- identifying the level of the audience (targeting to basic, advanced, clinical, management, education, or research nurses)
- developing the journal philosophy (focusing on nursing versus medical interventions)
- developing the writing style (using simple or complex sentence structure, suggesting wording preferences like "she/he," editing in or out words like "facilitated")
- selecting design styles (use of charts and pictures, length of articles, cover design)
- working with the publisher (meeting deadlines, length of the journal, number of issues per year)

The author's primary responsibility is to write the manuscript. Although this sounds easy to some editors, the difficulty is all too clear to the editor who both writes his or her own work and edits others' work. Authoring is not easy; it is hard work that requires multiple aspects:

- generating the idea (narrowing it, selecting from among several ideas)
- organizing the presentation (selecting headings, deciding on order of points)
- focusing on the reader (using examples of interest to the particular type of reader)
- using the journal format (selecting case study, research, or other formats)
- typing the manuscript in the journal style (recognizing different typing, reference, and chart styles)
- obtaining permissions (requesting permissions for pictures and copyrighted charts)
- checking accuracy (rechecking references, statements, quotations, and research data)

The nursing editor's and author's opinions agree on one aspect: what a book on writing should include. A book on writing for nurses should focus on the writing process, not the editing process. There are many books available on editing, but few that focus as well on the writing process as this one.

Donna Richards Sheridan and Donna Lee Dowdney help you as the author with a very practical focus on writing nursing manuscripts. The many checklists such as the ones on selecting a topic, analyzing a journal, developing a time schedule, and planning the writing will assist you in completing these difficult steps. New sections in this edition on advanced technology for writing assistance (computerized literature searches, CD-ROM databases, Internet Communication, and word processing) will speed your preparation and writing phases.

You will also find help in making critical decisions during the writing process. The authors include a review of the possible options for decisions during your writing, such as selecting the title, target journal, and organizational framework. These decision points are critical, each option creating a different manuscript.

For example, one often overlooked decision is selecting single or multiple authorship. The section on co-authoring is excellent, focusing on both options to help you decide if you will write alone or with a colleague. Deciding on co-authoring is not taken seriously enough by most authors, even though the decision frequently affects the quality of the manuscript. Authoring alone more likely results in a well-organized manuscript presenting a common philosophy and style throughout; co-authoring sometimes results in expanded perspectives and expertise. All editors fairly quickly recognize the importance of the author(s) making the decision on single or multiple authorship. Too frequently the editor is asked to mediate between co-authors who are no longer talking with one another or who each refuse to release a manuscript unless their name is listed as first author. Single or multiple authorship models can both be successful as long as you consider the advantages and disadvantages listed in this book and you use techniques to increase collaboration.

When you use the advice and exercises in this book, you will select a timely idea, target it to an interested journal and audience, organize it well, avoid the blocks to writing, write it to the journal's specific format, and enhance it with appropriate illustrations. Your manuscript will have a very good chance of acceptance and will require little developmental editing. Your manuscript will still need copyediting, a service provided by most nursing journal and book publishers. (Note: developmental editing involves reorganizing and rephrasing the manuscript; copyediting includes correcting grammar and editing to the publisher's style.)

Taking the risk of sounding obvious: a last word of advice. Use this book to help you to write the best manuscript you can and revise it until you have done your best; then let the editor edit. Editors like to edit and they like to be respected as editors. Do not be offended if the review board and editor have suggestions to strengthen your manuscript. Many nursing editors mention that 90% of the articles published were revised at least once before they were ready for publication. Save a little time and energy for this revision using the editor's suggestions. Very few authors can also edit their own material; they can edit others' materials, but they still need an editor for their own writing. It is possible that you are so close to the material you wrote that you cannot be an objective editor of that material. Fortunately, as the author of this foreword I will have the assistance of the book's and Springer Publishing Company's editors, and I gladly accept it. When you let the editor edit, your focus can turn to your next article or book project. Using the writing process in this book will assist you to develop not only one but many nursing manuscripts, making writing an ongoing process of communicating recent insights, opinions, observations, techniques, and research from your nursing practice.

SUZANNE HALL JOHNSON, MN, RN,C, CNS
Editor of Dimensions of Critical Care Nursing,
Nurse Author & Editor, and Recruitment, Retention & Restructuring Report
Director, Hall Johnson Communication, Inc.
Lakewood, Colorado

Foreword: A Nurse Author's Perspective

Twenty-five years ago I had my first article published in a nursing journal. It was also the first manuscript I ever submitted. Previously I had written only required papers for university courses and projects. Since that time I have published more than 110 articles, 3 books, several forewords, and half a dozen chapters in other authors' books. Also, I have written scripts for video and filmstrip productions, published several commercially successful self-learning packages, and even produced some marketing copy. This reasonably prolific output has not brought a great deal of money, but it has given me tremendous ego satisfaction and pleasure as well as highly valued visibility and credibility in my profession. It also, I hope, qualifies me to write a Foreword in this excellent book on the writing process.

Like anything worthwhile, writing requires effort, discipline, and practice. Writing is not something to be done casually or when the mood strikes. Writing must be planned and considered as a serious activity. As Ben Jonson says, "Who casts to write a living line, must sweat" *(To the Memory of My Beloved, the Author, Mr. William Shakespeare,* 1623). A good piece of writing is the result of a process similar to that required by any craft or art. Polishing, shaping, and reworking are very much a part of successful writing. Most writers believe their products or "babies" are beautiful and unique at birth, but like other people's children, such products, when first born, may only be ordinary ugly ducklings. A great effort is required to fulfill the promise and potential.

Although I have never taken a writing course nor was fortunate enough to have a book such as this one, I learned much and benefited greatly from my editors, colleagues, and other writers. Each critique and suggestion from an editor helped me improve my writing skills. As a result, although writing is still not "a piece of cake," it has become less traumatic. I cannot overemphasize the importance of good editing. Writers nurture ideas to reality, but editors make them readable and living by their conscientious pruning and shaping.

Every published manuscript, like every painting, is not a masterpiece, but each reflects its author's personality. Your writing is a reflection of your mind and spirit; it is an extension of you. Being published is a compliment granted to few. More manuscripts are rejected than are accepted. Not everyone is successful at writing. However, anyone can try. This book, which has certainly withstood the passages and changes of time, can be a tremendous help both in getting started and in continuing the process of writing. The authors have provided invaluable direction and practical advice and examples. They also have demonstrated the art of writing—they certainly practice what they preach.

Unlike other more physical activities, writing does not require youth or early training. You are never too old to try. As Benjamin Franklin, a most prolific and elderly writer, once said:

> If you would not be forgotten,
> As soon as you are dead and rotten,
> Either write things worth reading,
> or do things worth writing.
>
> POOR RICHARD'S ALMANAC, May 1738

And if all else fails, you can follow the advice of another well-known author, James Russell Lowell:

> Nature fits all her children with something to do
> He who would write and can't, can surely review.
>
> A FABLE FOR CRITICS, 1848

DOROTHY J. DEL BUENO EdD RN
Partner and Senior Consultant
Performance Management Services Inc.
Tustin, California

Preface

Many books begin as this one did—to meet a specific need that was not being met elsewhere. Nurses, the experts in nursing, need to share their expertise effectively by writing, not only for other nurses, but also for other health care professionals and the public. We worked with nurses who attempted to do this and found that they had many writer's blocks that our Writing and Marketing Process could prevent. This Process, developed to help nurses write, is a step-by-step alternative to facing a blank sheet of paper.

We developed our Process to include both the writing *and* marketing aspects, recognizing that while writing skills are important, focusing the writing toward a specific audience is the key to being published. We revised the Process continually as nurses used it in our Writing for Professional Publication Workshop at Stanford University Hospital. Participants in our workshops commented that they learned how to plan and organize their writing, stay focused on a topic, write clearly, and select appropriate target journals. One participant said, "The practical learning-through-doing process made it seem more probable that my ideas will become *real* articles." Many nurses have published their first articles using this Process.

One basic skill many nurses lack is the ability to organize their writing. We have developed this part of the Writing Process in detail because unorganized manuscripts are often difficult to salvage later. In all the writing workshops we have presented, we have spent a significant amount of time on the 10 steps within the organizing part of the Process. Participants have consistently indicated that this is helpful. Most participants had never used a Sun Diagram (see Figure 6.1) before the workshop, and most state that they would not write again without one.

We wrote this book because nurses attending our workshops asked for it—they wanted to continue using the Writing and Marketing Process after the workshop. Further, we are pleased to provide this Process to the greater nursing community so that more nurses may learn to share their expertise through writing for other health care professionals and for the public. The *American Journal of Nursing* awarded our book a "Book of the Year Award" in 1986. Since the publication of the first edition of this book in 1986, significant changes have occurred not only within nursing, but also within the publishing industry. One of these changes in publishing has resulted from increased use of electronic publishing, which has become one of the fastest changing areas in the communications field. Electronic publishing involves using personal computers, in combination with text, graphics, and page layout programs, to produce publication-quality documents. Electronic publishing has brought about the need for trained professionals who not only can communicate the content of their field, but who also can use the new technologies to do so. This newly revised book gives an overview of some of these changes and shows nurse writers how they can benefit.

Another new area the book addresses is the "information explosion." We show readers the possibilities of accessing online computerized databases, CD-ROM, and the Internet to retrieve and send information. We also updated the figures and tables and added many new ones to help nurses to write and publish articles in nursing.

1

Decide to Write

We wrote this book for nurses who want to write for professional publications. Editors want articles from practicing nurses. Whether you practice in clinical, educational, administrative, or research areas, you have the nursing and health care information and knowledge editors are seeking. You have the expertise and experience your colleagues are eager to read about. "Clinical nurses know what works, what doesn't, and how to trouble shoot clinical problems. Yet many hesitate to put their ideas into manuscript form" (Sheridan, 1994a, p. 1).

Nurses need to write about nursing and patient care. As Donna Diers, Dean and Professor of the Yale School of Nursing said: "That is the field we know best, those of us who practice, and nobody else can write about it as we can. . . . For some reason, it seems very hard for nurses to think about writing about what they know best, and know better than anyone else in the world, and that's patient care" (Diers, 1981, p. 8).

Nursing needs writers.

You completed that project, you chaired that committee, you wrote those standards, you solved that problem. Now tell your peers! Nurses want to read "how-to" stories and you can learn to tell yours in the nursing literature. . . . Now is the time to get that information out of your head and onto paper. The sense of accomplishment achieved through publishing is surpassed only by the incorporation of your contributions to the nursing literature. We must "profess" in the nursing literature in order for nursing to be a "profession" (Sheridan, 1994a, p. 1)

Yet, because of a busy schedule or lack of writing experience, your important ideas are often not written down. "Prospective writers are finding it harder to write than ever before. Fear of rejection is not the greatest problem anymore; instead, the obstacle is finding the time and energy to write" (Johnson, 1995, p. 4).

Writing is hard work, and you may not be convinced that writing for professional publications is worth your time. Mundt (1977) observed that nurses as a group see themselves as doers rather than as thinkers or planners: "While other professionals philosophize and synthesize, nurses keep busy with direct care activities and do not take time out to express themselves in writing" (p. 6).

WHY WRITE FOR PROFESSIONAL PUBLICATION?

Many reasons for writing for professional publication have been shared in the nursing literature. "The effective use of publication skills can promote interdisciplinary communication, bring about improved patient care, and enhance professional, personal, and organizational growth" (Klarman & Mateo, 1994, p. 35). An overview of comments from successful nurse writers is reviewed below.

Advancing the Profession

Vernice D. Ferguson, as Deputy Assistant Chief Medical Director for Nursing Programs and Director, Nursing Service, Veterans Administration, wrote:

> Generally a profession is known by its societal service mandate, its distinctive educational preparation to provide that service, and authority of its practice. Such authority is derived from knowledge. Professional persons "profess" to practice from the best available knowledge as they provide service to people. That knowledge must be generated constantly, published regularly, and utilized always as professional nurses practice. (Ferguson, 1984, p. 35)

Margretta M. Styles, former Dean of the School of Nursing, University of California at San Francisco, and President of the International Council of Nurses reiterates that "The primary reason to publish is because the future of the profession depends on it." She elaborates by saying that the aphorism of "publish or perish" is true not only for individuals, but also for disciplines. "Scholarly productivity is a natural, inescapable standard for survival for individuals who make up the profession . . . scholarly means that we possess profound knowledge on a particular subject. And the means of scholarly communication is publication" (Styles, 1978, pp. 28–32).

Scholarly journals represent professionalism in a discipline. *Image* and *Nursing Forum* indicate that nursing values scholarly inquiry and investigation. "Nurses are increasingly assuming responsibility for writing the articles in their own journals, instead of looking to physicians or members of other disciplines to write about nursing for them" (Hayter, 1984, p. 362).

Writing for publication is not easy, but if nursing is to grow and become recognized for its true value in the health care community, nurses must seek opportunities for enhancing their writing skills.

Authorship by nurses requires commitment. Since nursing is a dynamic process, professional knowledge and skills improve and advance as society and technology dictate. In nurses' daily practice in the clinical setting, they observe, evaluate, adapt, and recommend. Thus, it is vital to nursing that nurses share their knowledge with peers through writing. "Advancement of the nursing profession requires it. It is one route to nursing excellence" (Salome, 1983, p. 51).

Sharing New Perspectives and Experiences

One of the great opportunities of life is sharing your experiences and philosophy with others. Your professional nursing experiences are important to others for the growth and development of the nursing profession. By writing about these experiences you are sharing in the promotion of better patient care and inspiring students and colleagues who will benefit from the exchange. (Coraluzzo, 1977, p. 55)

Writing for professional publications gives nurses recognition for their health care contributions. Through writing, you, as a practicing nurse, may offer new ideas about approaches to old situations, make suggestions for innovative directions in nursing, and present a unique perspective on current health care issues. Kolin and Kolin (1980) pointed out that "The nurse who wants to share something worthwhile helps not only the profession as a whole, but also individual practitioners . . . Broad-scope journals such as the *American Journal of Nursing* or *Nursing* number their readers in hundreds of thousands" (p. 165).

You can share your experiences with other nurses by explaining new and useful clinical procedures; sharing helpful nursing care plans; suggesting methods of cost containment; or educating colleagues in nursing applications and adaptations to new technologies. You may challenge or support the usefulness of some nursing models, concepts, and theories; report research you have completed; or describe a solution you worked out to a problem with a difficult patient.

Professional publications require new ideas and authors to survive. Because professional publications exist to serve the profession, new ideas are essential to stimulate professional growth. Journals keep nurses abreast of changing medical and nursing practices, challenge the utility of nursing models, integrated curricula, and concepts of practice, and teach procedures for patient care. Sister Rosemary Donley wrote, "I believe that a journal regardless of its sponsorship should be a critical force and forum for questioning beliefs and advancing knowledge" (Donley, 1982, p. 68).

Reporting Research and the Changing Status of Nursing

JoAnn Brooks-Brunn offers tips on writing a research-based manuscript, stating: "Written communication of research in the form of a journal manuscript is an important part of the research process" (Brooks-Brunn, 1991, p. 1). There is an old adage in research that the research is not complete until it is reported.

Joyce Black, MSN, RNC, of *Plastic Surgical Nursing*, discussed each aspect of writing for publication. Her article, "Writing for Publication: Advice to Potential Authors," includes tips on generating topics, writing first drafts, editing, and submitting to a journal (Black, 1992).

Improving Health Care

Patients can benefit from nurses' writing and sharing ideas to improve the quality and cost-effectiveness of health care. "That writing has to come from those who know it most dearly and daily, and they are the most qualified for that kind of writing. The perceptions of the new staff nurse and the clinical wisdom of the veteran must somehow get out of their heads and onto the paper, for we need their words so much" (Diers, 1981, p. 8).

Enhancing Nursing's Image

Nurses have been reticent to explain to the public and to other professionals the knowledge and competencies they need to function in their various roles and settings. Nurses possess information and knowledge to share with each other. We can share our successes and failures with other nurses as we write for professional publications.

Increasing Chances of Promotion

Writing for professional publications not only helps you advance professionally, but also meets publication requirements in academic settings.

Growing Professionally

Writing may lead to opportunities to present speeches and workshops. Or, conversely, the content of speeches and workshops may be shared with your colleagues through writing. Either way, writing offers the opportunity for professional growth, personal recognition, and enhanced prestige.

Receiving Personal Rewards

Professional writing provides personal as well as professional satisfaction because writers are inspired to preserve their thoughts and ideas for future reference. The mark of a civilization is its written records that reveal people's lifestyles and works in subsequent generations. Thus, people write so that their thoughts, ideas, and feelings are not forgotten; they want to extend their teachings beyond their immediate environments through articles and books.

> I want to share my knowledge base with others interested in emergency nursing. I want to preserve my synthesized body of knowledge systematically for those practitioners with less experience or perhaps a different type of exposure from mine. Writing forces me to think critically and to organize my thoughts carefully. It insists that I research and document and assume accountability for what I am conveying. It represents a starting point for others who wish to build on what I have learned and allows them to profit from my mistakes. (Barber, 1980, p. 45)

A personal benefit from writing is the process involved in sorting out your ideas and organizing your thoughts. As you write, you will critique the practice of nursing, ask questions, and affect future practice. Seeing your ideas in print gives you satisfaction that you are contributing to others' practice and perhaps bettering patient care. Your writing can address human experiences with compassionate realism and clinical expertise. Sister Rosemary Donley, during her tenure as Dean of Nursing at the Catholic University of America, said that the primary reward she derives from writing is personal joy and satisfaction (Sheridan & Dowdney, 1984).

WHY NURSE LEADERS WRITE

For the first edition of this book, we sent surveys to a group of selected prominent nurse authors, a group of randomly chosen nurse authors, and a group of nursing journal editors. We asked selected prominent nurse authors, "What is your primary reward derived from writing?" Most of these authors are still writing and publishing. All of their responses are timeless:

GENROSE J. ALFANO: I write to share information—but mostly to try to influence thinking of others!

JUNE T. BAILEY: I write to assist students and nurses to understand difficult concepts and theories.

BARBARA J. BROWN: I write to get rid of frustrations and because of requests from others. It's usually fun, creative self-expression.

LUTHER CHRISTMAN: I write for clarification of my own thoughts.

DOROTHY J. DEL BUENO: I write for visibility/credibility.

DONNA DIERS: I write for the hell of it. The fun of it. To think up new ways of saying things, play with words and ideas, get clear about something.

VERNICE FERGUSON: I enjoy speaking and writing and recognize that writing assures permanence. Positive feedback is a factor as well.

M. JANICE NELSON: I enjoy writing—it's an excellent outlet for formulating ideas, backing them up, developing logic to an idea, etc.

BARBARA STEVENS/BARNUM: It has changed with age. Originally, it is terribly exciting to think that you said something important enough to merit publication. Later, you write just because you "have to," i.e., have something that you feel you must share.

MARGRETTA M. STYLES: I write to stimulate my creative edge.

RHEBA DE TORNYAY: It is a way of life for me. I love to write ideas and views and I couldn't feel like a professional without writing.

DUANE D. WALKER: I write for publicity and the satisfaction of meeting a goal.

HELEN YURA: I write to influence nursing and nursing practice in a positive way.

MARY LLOYD ZUSY: I write because I have ideas and like to share them. The chief reward is the feeling that what I write may make a difference.

Sister M. Paschala Noonan (1961) said,

I could mention many reasons why I write. I write to provide a Christmas surprise for somebody I love when I have nothing else to give but my gift of words. I write to express heartfelt gratitude to the school of nursing where I trained. . . . Sometimes I write to sing of people who capture my imagination—some patient, nurse, or doctor—or to ease a need or an emotional hunger. I write to help young mothers because they needed help when everyone else is too busy to bother with them . . . I write to get money to help pay for an incubator for our nursery, or maybe to get a wheel chair for a sick Sister. And sometimes I write because something inside of me gnaws until I get it on paper. . . . Lately, I find myself writing because of a gripe. So many articles appear in popular magazines giving a distorted picture of the nursing profession. It's time the nurses who know that profession better than anyone else speak for themselves. (pp. 246–248)

Finally, Margretta M. Styles wrote "The Thrill of it All" (1978), a classic, in *Image*:

1. It is a tremendous thrill for those who express themselves in ideas, rather than clay or watercolors or music or bridges, to see the embodiment of those ideas in published form. This is the kind of physical extension of one's mind—and a possible form of immortality.
2. It is a tremendous thrill to discover that one's published work has been applied in improving professional practice.
3. It is a tremendous thrill to learn that one's published work is the basis for teaching and learning.
4. It is a tremendous thrill to see the evidence that one's published work has stimulated and contributed to the work of others in the discipline or even in other disciplines.
5. It is a tremendous thrill to find one's circle of professional friends and one's scope of professional influence widening and widening, across the nation, around the world.
6. It is a tremendous thrill to be invited to speak as an expert at a national or international scientific meeting.
7. It is a tremendous thrill to be recognized for one's published work through professional and academic honors and awards.
8. It is a tremendous thrill to be recognized and rewarded by promotion and tenure in academic institutions known for the rigor of their scholarship.
9. And undeniably, it's a tremendous thrill to receive additional income and to increase one's creature comforts as a result of the salary raises which accompany promotion and as a result of the royalties from publication.

However, following the thrill of it all is the pain in publishing:

1. There is the pain involved in the discipline, discipline, discipline, discipline of writing.
2. There is the pain involved in squeezing in the extra hours for creative activity between the crushing blocks of practice and teaching responsibility, the pain of housing a creative mind in a fatigued or restless body.
3. There is the pain of methodically and systematically searching out and documenting one's sources, writing and rewriting and rewriting.
4. There is the pain of criticism of one's cherished ideas.
5. There is the pain of finding the right publisher, of waiting patiently for his decision.

6. There is the pain of rejection. The pain of picking up and starting again. (pp. 28–32)

She concludes, "But, not to publish is an aching nothingness in a part of one's professional soul" (p. 32).

WHY DO PEOPLE READ PROFESSIONAL PUBLICATIONS?

People read professional publications to learn about new developments, new concepts, new approaches to existing practices, and specialized information. They want to become better informed through new interpretations and opinions. Readers want to learn details about new developments in the field so that they can become more effective as professionals. In addition, they want to learn about professional activities and obtain specialized information about products.

YOU ARE QUALIFIED TO WRITE

Within your scope of practice are many topics, and you are qualified to write about them. You can write about situations, problems and solutions, and patient cases in your current work setting. Writing about what is familiar to you brings a fresh, reality-based approach to your articles that appeals to editors.

For example, June L. Stark in *Nursing '94* wrote "Interpreting B.U.N./ Creatinine Levels" (1994). As a critical care nurse educator, she explained what these nitrogenous wastes reveal about your patient's renal status. Although the author obviously spent some time researching the current literature on nitrogenous waste, she had selected a topic familiar to her daily practice. The benefits are cyclic; her practice in this specialty will enrich her article. The information gathered and organized on this topic will enhance her knowledge and enrich her practice.

WRITER'S BLOCK

What keeps nurses from writing? One major barrier is writer's block, a writer's occupational hazard. Procrastination is a major symptom of writer's block.

Lawrence Block, author of more than 100 published novels, shared some fears that block his writing: that he would not get it written; that he did not have enough to say on the topic; that the column would lack substance; that he would repeat himself; that nobody would be interested; that someone would write him a nasty letter about it; and that he would not be able to think of what to write the following month. After he listed other fears, Block concluded, "It's useful though, to root out and list these more general fears about writing. Once you've found out what your fears are, you can devise affirmations to reverse them" (Block, 1984, p. 52).

To help avoid procrastination and build a positive attitude toward your writing, keep in mind the time-tested advice of successful writers:

- Use past success to bolster you: you *have* completed writing tasks before; understand that you *will* this time.
- Avoid the trap of thinking that everything you write should be either effortless or impossibly difficult.
- Remember that the sooner you get to work, the sooner you'll be finished (Alred, Oliu, & Brusaw, 1992, pp. 204–205).

"Analysis paralysis" is another symptom of writer's block. This malady affects writers who agonize over the first paragraph, the title, proper construction, grammar, and punctuation. A related problem is becoming a "pendant"—a person who makes needless display of learning or who insists upon the importance of trifling points of scholarship. Pedantic writers tend to lapse into unnecessary detail and jargon and sound rather boring and labored.

Frequently writer's block results from fear that editors will reject ideas or that others will find fault. Edwina McConnell responded to the question, "Why don't more nurses write for publications?":

> People don't write because they're afraid. I believe that's why a lot of nurses don't write nursing care plans, because when you put something down on paper it's there for everybody to see. It's there for physicians to see if they look at the Kardex and it's there for your peers to see. No one wants to appear foolish—that's the fear. They can't criticize it, if you don't put it down in writing. So I do think it is, in part, fear of being laughed at, fear of being wrong, and fear of not knowing the right words to use. Writing is a creation of our own and we tend to think of it as an extension of ourselves. We take criticism personally. (Baloff, 1982, p. 42)

Overcoming Writer's Block

To deal with writer's block. try to determine what is blocking your writing. If it is lack of confidence, read articles on topics that interest you. Do you ever feel that you could have written a better article than the ones you see in print? Talk with colleagues about the topics on which you want to write. This will help to clarify your thoughts, which will help you to see the merit of your ideas.

We asked selected nurse authors (Sheridan & Dowdney, 1984): "What writing blocks have you had and how have you overcome them?" Perhaps their experiences are similar to yours . . . and perhaps their suggestions are just what you need.

GENROSE J. ALFANO: I don't like detail, and rewriting—I suspect "Indolence" is a major problem! I need to feel what I'm writing can make a difference and . . . I need a deadline.

JUNE T. BAILEY: I am a perfectionist and at times rewrite articles too many times.

BARBARA J. BROWN: I take a long walk on the beach to clear my head. Read the subject matter. Sleep. Reapproach the subject, gather information.

RHEBA DE TORNYAY: If it doesn't flow, I stop for the day.

DONNA DIERS: Usually, the block is trying to find the hook to hang the piece on and that simply requires more thinking or talking with somebody. Sometimes, I just start a paper and type whatever comes to mind and then figure out where it's going and what's wrong with it. "Writing oneself clear."

LOUCINE M. HUCKABAY: English is a second language to me. After I write a research article or a book, I hire an editor to correct my grammar and style to fit the journal or publisher. It costs lots of money.

M. JANICE NELSON: Mostly, just getting started. My way is to start writing—anything. Once the ideas begin to gel and follow some logical order, then go back and start "the cleaning-up process."

BARBARA STEVENS/BARNUM: Often my publishers will want new editions of a book just when I would prefer to do something else. The thought of royalties finally drives me to new editions.

HELEN YURA: Finding time to write while working full time at positions with a lot of responsibility. Planning ahead is the solution and having a superb coauthor with whom to work.

A common theme in these selected nurse authors' blocks is lack of time, yet they are finding the time. One successful nurse author said, "I don't really like deadlines (even when I set them). But one does what one has to do. Once I start, it's all OK." Realize that you will always be busy and have more than enough things to take up your time. If you wait until you have the time you think you need, you will never write.

In *Writer's Digest*, Robyn Carr observed that

> There are a lot of reasons why people who want to write don't, and amazingly, only one of them is time. People don't write today because they won't have time to continue tomorrow . . . People don't write because they aren't ready . . . And people don't write because they're scared that when they do write, it won't be good enough. People don't write because they only have an hour . . . Or they work all day to get all their 'obligations' taken care of so they can finally write guilt free, only to find themselves exhausted and brainless. People don't write because someone is going to interrupt them any second, or they don't write because everyone in the family has helped them clear the time and now the pressure is too intense. (Carr, 1995, p. 28)

She goes on to recommend that if you want to write, find out where the time is. Make writing a priority. Let some things go. Alter the way you do things. Organize. Don't try to do everything and be everything to everyone. She concludes:

> After examining your schedule, your priorities and obligations, is there simply *no time left?* Is there nothing to trade off except sleep? Is there nothing about the way you do things that can be changed or compromised or eliminated? You're simply booked up, from morning till night? If so, then I submit to you that you haven't quite decided that writing is terribly important to you. And trust me on this one—if it isn't all that important, you'll be wasting your time. Writing is one of those things you have to want . . . and you have to want it bad. (Carr, 1995, p. 28)

When you start with the topic that most appeals to you, stay with it until you see it in print. Then, similar to the amateur golfer who hits only one good shot, you will be back trying again.

Find a place to write where you can keep your reference books, files, paper, and writing tools. Most important, designate a time to be writing in that place—early morning or after work or late evening . . . whatever time works for you. But be sure the time is regularly scheduled, and follow through on doing some piece of work during that committed time. Make writing an important priority and set goals for yourself—what you want to achieve and when you want to achieve it.

To understand and improve your writing style and grammatical constructions, consult writing books in the library and publications such as *Writer's Digest, The Writer, Freelance Writer's Report, Technical Communication, The Quill, Writer's Journal,* and *Writer's Connection* (See Appendix 1). Join writers' associations (See Appendix 2) or local journal clubs.

To avoid analysis paralysis, recognize that hours of data collection and library searching may not be necessary for the particular article you want to write. You can approach necessary library work efficiently by differentiating between articles that need an entire review of the literature and articles that need only a brief review on a specific topic in a few targeted journals.

Information may also be available as direct quotes from your colleagues who are experts on the topic. Computer abstracts may give you some of the information you need or lead you to key articles on your topic. Your own practice, surveys, or research may also efficiently add to your database. Also, learn to use the library effectively and efficiently. Chapter 5 gives more ideas about gathering information.

Write regularly in order to form a habit of writing. "The writing habit, unlike smoking, is extremely easy to break. We can feel truly addicted, to the point where if we fail to sit down at the typewriter regularly, we experience psychological, even physiological discomfort. And yet, that failure over even a brief period of time usually results in a quick dissipation of the energies that have been providing our motivation" (Jacobs, 1985, p. 8).

Writer's workshops, classes, and conferences can help you learn how others overcame writing obstacles and blocks, identify markets for your writing, and increase your writing skills. "Writers are people who never stop examining and learning, and university and college extensions are like wonderlands for the curious" (Wilson, 1983, p. 58).

Workshops are available from coast to coast. Often writing workshops are offered as a part of a national conference. Sheridan (co-author of this book) often teaches at Mosby-Yearbook Resource Applications workshops with numerous participants publishing post conference. Don't miss opportunities to attend these to start on your article and, even better, to talk with editors. Increasingly, writing courses are being offered in nursing academia: "We are confident that integrating a specific methodology for writing instruction into a nursing course has produced important gains for both students and faculty. . . . We have learned, and our students have become better thinkers and writers" (Pinkava & Haviland, 1984, p. 272)

In addition, workshops are often offered at adult education programs and community colleges. Dowdney (co-author of this book) teaches regularly at De Anza College in California. Look in current nursing journals and community fliers for other writing workshops to attend.

Writing conferences for nonhealth care professionals are helpful. Besides community colleges, professional associations such as the American Medical Writers Association, Council of Biology Editors, the Society for Technical Communication, European Association of Science Editors, and the Association for Business Communication offer writing workshops.

Writer's Digest publishes an annual list of scores of writer's conferences held in the United States and internationally. Most conferences are structured around workshops, lectures, and individual coaching. Writer's conferences also offer opportunities to meet other writers, editors, publishers, and agents. In deciding which conference to attend, consider each of the following points:

- Review the conference objectives to determine whether they meet your needs.
- Evaluate the cost/benefit to you regarding registration fee, distance, length of conference, accommodations, and workshop content.
- Evaluate opportunities for professional networking with colleagues and editors.
- Select speakers with excellent writing and teaching credentials.
- Ask other nurses for recommendations of good writing conferences.
- Determine the availability of a one-to-one consultation on a specific manuscript (submit ahead if possible).

THE WRITING PROCESS

We have developed and integrated parts of The Writing Process into a clear, straightforward model, The Writing Process Model. Through this Process, you too can translate your valuable information into a published article. The Writing Process Model shows the specific steps you can take to write an article for publication in nursing. We have written this book around The Writing Process Model (See Figure 1-1). Each chapter is a step in The Writing Process Model.

Chapter One, "Decide to Write," reviews many reasons nurse authors write, as well as what readers want in professional publications. The chapter also explores the problem of writer's block and suggests how to overcome it. The Writing Process, the core of this book, is introduced. It is the key to moving from your idea to your published manuscript.

Chapter Two, "Generate Ideas," suggests several sources for writing ideas and indicates topics on which nursing journal editors prefer articles. Then the chapter presents guidelines for selecting topics.

Chapter Three, "Develop a Plan," addresses the advantages and disadvantages of collaboration gleaned from the insights of successful nurse authors. The chapter helps you create a writing plan that includes the organizing idea, the purpose of the manuscript, the organizing framework, working title, theme, development method, target audience and journal,

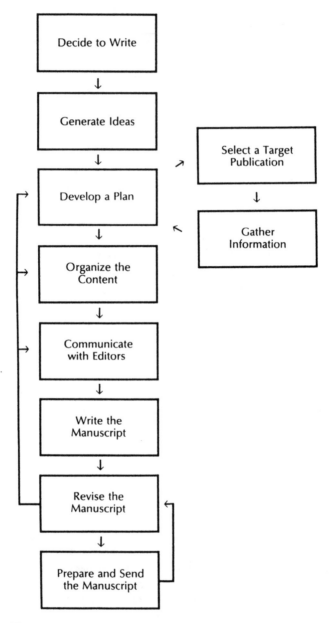

Figure 1.1. The writing and marketing process (© 1983, Sheridan & Dowdney).

and a time schedule for completing the manuscript. The plan details the steps of The Writing Process.

Chapter Four, "Select a Target Publication," shows you how to analyze publications for journal theme, audience, style and tone, organizing framework, viewpoint, and timeliness. The chapter also addresses writing for nonhealth care markets and presents the Target Journal Selection and Tracking Form and the Target Journal Marketing and Analysis Form.

Chapter Five, "Gather Information," explains how to keep up to date in nursing, ideas for setting up a manuscript critique group, and how to initiate a library search. It indicates databases for computer searches and techniques for using CD-ROM and The Internet. It also presents interviewing strategies and techniques as well as the advantages of networking with other writers.

Chapter Six, "Organize the Content," presents steps for organizing the content, including focusing the topic, listing and grouping the ideas, finding the framework, and creating and revising the diagrams and outlines.

Chapter Seven, "Communicate with Editors," deals with initiating communication with editors through query letters, telephone calls, meetings at conferences, and sending complete manuscripts. The chapter also presents types of leads to use in query letters and articles, and acceptance and rejection of manuscripts as experienced by successful nurse authors.

Chapter Eight, "Write the Manuscript," tells how to prepare to write and how to select a title and lead. Then it takes you through the process of developing paragraphs, topic sentences, and transitions. It also shows you how to select computer hardware and software for word processing. The chapter describes plagiarism and libel, and concludes with instructions in preparing your manuscript's final draft.

Chapter Nine, "Revise the Manuscript," reviews basic grammatical terms and concepts and reveals common pitfalls along with strategies to avoid them. The chapter also reviews types of sentences and presents principles for improving writing.

Chapter Ten, "Prepare and Send the Manuscript," deals with format, content, and readability. It describes required permissions and procedures for obtaining them. Peer review and refereed publications are also discussed.

Appendix 1 lists publications of interest to writers.

Appendix 2 lists selected writing and literary associations.

Appendix 3 presents information about professional nursing journals.

Using the Writing Process, you can proceed through an efficient sequence to produce a published article by completing a series of techniques that "pull you through" the Process. You never have to face a blank sheet of paper, not knowing where to begin.

We have arranged the information so that activities are integrated with didactic material to help you develop skills in thinking and writing while increasing your knowledge about how to write. Through this step-by-step, skill-building approach, workshop participants and individuals we coached have become proficient at each step of the process with resultant strong, clear, well-organized articles, and you can, too.

Each time you use this book to guide your writing, the writing process becomes easier. After you write a few articles, you will be able to move more quickly through the steps at which you are most skillful. Slow progress at any step in the Process may indicate a need for further skill building in that area. The book will continually guide you through that difficult step to meet your individual learning needs about writing.

Although writing is a skill that improves with practice, writing skills alone are insufficient for having your article published. The skills involved in "selling" your manuscript to "buyers" in the nursing market (editors) are also essential. Many nurses who are novice writers have good ideas about article topics. After they spend much time writing, however, they send their manuscripts to journals only to receive rejection letters from editors. For this reason, marketing concepts have been included throughout this book. Communicating with an editor is vital and needs to be integrated throughout the writing of the manuscript. Otherwise your well-written manuscript will be rejected. It may sit forever on a shelf, never reaching the publication goal of The Writing Process.

One predictable reason for manuscripts being rejected is that writers do not investigate which publications are most appropriate for a particular article. In this book, you will learn about selecting a target market for your manuscript. This will substantially increase your chances of having your articles accepted for publication.

For example, if you had sent a manuscript to *Nursing Economics* in April of 1994 on funding levels for advanced practice nurses, it would be obvious to the editor that you had not looked at the previous month's issue; otherwise, you would have seen an article on this topic and known this journal was not likely to repeat an article on this subject again so soon. Or perhaps you send an article to *Heart & Lung, The Journal of Critical Care,* on traumatic lung injury, a topic in which the editors had great interest, but since you failed to include a transmittal letter, which this journal requires before the editors review any manuscript, your article is returned. In the interim, the journal receives someone else's similar article that includes the required transmittal letter. If this latter article is accepted, your article is no longer of value to this publication. *Heart & Lung* actually provides a 13-item checklist for authors along with two pages of guidelines. When journals dedicate this much space to author guidelines, they expect compliance in submitted manuscripts.

In addition, nursing journal editors reject articles that deal primarily with medical procedures. For nursing journals, the topic must deal with *nursing* implications or *nursing* care related to the medical procedure. Elinor S. Schrader, former editor of *Association of Operating Room Nurses Journal* (AORN), and mentor to many nurse authors, once said that one of the primary reasons for rejecting articles is that the "articles are *medical*, not *nursing*." She went on to say that while it is acceptable to give some medical or nonnursing background, "articles must be written primarily with a nursing focus including such information as nursing process, nursing actions, and nursing innovations." (Sheridan, 1982, p. 11).

Even articles addressing very technical or physiological subjects need to be written with a nursing focus if the article is for a nursing journal.

A rejection letter is also predictable for the nurse who sends a clinical manuscript entitled, "Stat Lab Tests Dictate the Immediate Nursing Care of the Hemodialysis Patient" to an administrative journal such as the *Journal of Nursing Administration* or sends "Elizabeth Had Anorexia Nervosa: A Case Study" to the *Journal of Nursing Research.* Journals need to be thoroughly examined for the type of article they include and the topics they cover.

Although the above nurse authors may have had useful information to share, they did not select the appropriate journals. Journal editors target their publications for a specific audience and continually assess what that market will buy. They look for manuscripts to meet their readers' identified needs.

If you want to know what editors are seeking, simply ask. They are happy to share information about their publication needs in writer's guidelines. Writer's guidelines are written communications from editors/publishers to writers specifying the purpose and audience of the journal, selection of appropriate manuscript topics of current interest to their publication, and the preferred manuscript format including style, number of words, deadlines, references, and footnotes. Nursing journal editors usually make writer's guidelines available when you send an addressed, stamped envelope. Some also offer sample copies of their publications. Guidelines and samples will help you develop and send articles to the appropriate publications.

Writer's guidelines may also be found in journals. For example, *The Journal of Continuing Education in Nursing* (JCEN) contains the following information for authors: editor's name, number of required duplicate manuscripts, statement of the journal's purpose, manuscript preparation guidelines including typing format, style, references, releases and acknowledgments, requirement for a letter of transmittal, and a description of the review process. *Nursing Management* guidelines are found in the journal. This journal's "Information for Authors" footnote is typical. In small print under the listing of the editorial board (or under subscription information) is a succinct description of how to submit a manuscript, including a brief purpose statement. In *Nursing Management* the author information reads: "This journal considers original essays that explore, from a managerial perspective, issues concerning nursing practice, operations and environments. Texts should not exceed 15 double-spaced with an inch margin, 8½ x 11 typed pages, two copies which may be accompanied by references, bibliography and exhibits cleared for publication." The address follows along with an offer for detailed guidelines upon request. A final sentence details the expectations of the cover letter requesting inclusion of the author's name, credentials, occupational affiliations, address, phone and succinct description of the scope of the topic. Although not as thorough as the author information in *JCEN,* it is sufficient to knowledgeably submit a manuscript.

If you write or call for guidelines, some editors are especially helpful. In addition to sharing publishing needs with you, some editors will also share information about your specific topic and provide direction for developing the article before you write it.

How to write and how to work with an editor are the key factors integrated into The Writing Process. Thus, the model presents a process. "A writer is not so much someone who has something to say as he is someone who has found a process that will bring about new things he would not have thought of if he had not started to say them" (Stafford, 1982).

To get the most out of this book, select a topic on which you want to write and develop your topic through each stage of the process as you read through each chapter. Try the techniques presented with each step of The Writing Process—these will help to clarify your thoughts and build your writing skills as you write your article.

EXERCISE

Richard VanDeWeghe (1983) described several writing models. One type, the discovery model, involves nonstop writing without concern for structure, coherence, or correction—the writer follows digressions wherever they lead. This model has the disadvantages of taking too much time, of being a chaotic, disorganized process, and of leaving the writer with a wealth of unstructured material. However, one great advantage to the model is the notion of free flow. Free flow writing is a technique in which your pen follows your flow of thoughts. You need a pad of paper and a few pencils. Then you begin writing whatever comes into your head. "Keep thinking. Keep writing." You can even write that you "don't know what to write" . . . but don't stop writing.

On a pad of paper, try free-flow writing to describe your experience with writer's block. Include all details of the experience such as times when you can't write, feelings about writing, types of interruptions, and excuses for not writing. You could begin with, "I have writer's block when . . ." . Include workable ideas that you can use to prevent or break through your individual writing blocks.

REFERENCES

Alred, G. J., Oliu, W. E., & Brusaw, C. T. (1992). *The professional writer.* New York: St. Martin's Press.

Baloff, E. (1982, November). Interview: Edwina A. McConnell. *Today's OR Nurse, 4*(9), 38–44, 60–63.

Barber, J. (1980, September/October). The emergency nurse as writer. *Journal of Emergency Nursing,* p. 45.

Black, J. (1992). Writing for publication: Advice to potential authors. *Plastic Surgical Nursing, 12,* 155–158.

Block, L. (1984, August). Fear of writing. *Writer's Digest, 52.*

Brooks-Brunn, J. (1991). Tips on writing a research-based manuscript: The review of literature. *Nurse Author and Editor,* 1–3.

Campbell, C. (1983, September 14). Nurses in journalism. *Nursing Mirror, 52.*

Carr, R. (1995, June). How to make time to write. *Writer's Digest,* p. 28.

Coraluzzo, K. (1977). How to develop your natural writing skills. *The Journal of Continuing Education in Nursing, 8*(1), 55.

Diers, D. (1981). Why write? Why publish? *Image, 13*(1), 8.

Donley, R. (1982). The role of nursing journals? *Image, 14*(3), 68.

Ferguson, V. D. (1984). Finding meaning and direction. *Image, 16*(2), 35.

Hayter, J. (1984). Institutional sources of articles published in 13 nursing journals, 1978–1982. *Nursing Research, 33*(6), 362.

Hints for contributors. (1984). *RN, 14*(6), 96.

Jacobs, H. B. (1985, January). New York market letter. *Writer's Digest, 8.*

Johnson, S. H. (1981). Nurses' writing blocks. *Journal of Continuing Education in Nursing, 12*(6), 14–17.

Johnson, S. H. (1995). Getting clinical authors—even during healthcare reform. *Nurse Author and Editor, 5,* 4, 7–8.

Jones, I. H. (1984). From inspiration to publication. *Nursing Mirror, 158*(7), 44.

Klarman, K. L., & Mateo, M. A. (1994). Promoting the development of nurses' presentation and publication skills. *Health Care Supervisor, 12,* 35–40.

Kolin, P. C., & Kolin, J. L. (1980). *Professional writing for nurses in education, practice, and research.* St. Louis: C. V. Mosby.

Mundt, E. (1977). Why don't nurses write? *Nurse Educator, 2*(2), 6.

Noonan, M. P. (1961). An irresistible urge to write. *Nursing Outlook, 9*(4), 246–248.

Pinkava, B. P., & Haviland, C. P. (1984). Teaching writing and thinking skills. *Nursing Outlook, 32*(5), 272.

Salome, P. B. (1983). Program for success: Is writing the key to advancement? *Today's OR Nurse, 4*(12), 20–22, 51.

Sheridan, D. R. (1982). AORN editor recruits nursing articles. *Stanford Nurse, 4*(4), 11.

Sheridan, D. R. (1994a). Motivating clinical nurses to write for publication. *Nurse Author and Editor, 4*, 1–2.

Sheridan, D. R. (1994b). Write right now: A commitment, an idea, a plan. *Nursing Staff Development Insider, 3*, 6.

Sheridan, D. R., & Dowdney, D. L. (1984). *Survey of selected nurse authors.* Unpublished manuscript.

Stafford, W. (1982, February). Writing the Australian crawl. *The Writer,* 17.

Stark, J. L. (1994). Interpreting B.U.N./creatinine levels. *Nursing 94, 24,* 58–61.

Styles, M. M. (1978). Why publish? *Image, 10*(2), 28–32.

VanDeWeghe, R. (1983). Writing models, versatile writers. *Journal of Business Communication, 20*(1), 13–23.

Wilson, J. M. (1983, March). The west market report. *Writer's Digest,* 58.

2

Generate Ideas

> There is one thing stronger than all the
> armies in the world: and that is an idea
> whose time has come.
>
> —*Victor Hugo*

All practicing nurses are potential authors. Surrounding you at work are numerous ideas that you could develop into manuscripts. "I am always thinking of materials suitable for publication as I go about my work routine," said a nurse author from Portland.

"First you have to have an idea," said Mary Jane Zusy, as editor of *The Maryland Nurse*. "I write because I have ideas and like to share them" (Sheridan & Dowdney, 1984). You cannot write until you have something to write about.

If you already have several topics about which to write, this chapter will help you select the first topic to develop. If you do not have a topic yet, this chapter suggests many sources of topic ideas.

IDEAS FOR WRITING

Ideas are everywhere. You can develop an inquiring mind that will allow good manuscript ideas to emerge from what others see as everyday situations. You can begin to ask questions such as, "Why did this happen?" or "What caused this problem?" or "Why did everything go so smoothly this time?"

Watch for ideas during discussions with colleagues, as you read news articles, as you develop care plans and workshops, and as you solve administrative problems. Keep your ears open for new procedures and approaches to care or new solutions to old problems.

Work Environment

Looking in your work environment for article ideas makes good sense because you should only write about topics with which you are familiar. In our survey of selected nurse authors, Sarah E. Archer, then Professor at the University of California, San Francisco, said, "Have something to say, know what you're talking about from your own experience, know your audience and talk to them. Don't be erudite for erudition's sake. Write for people in such a way that they can use the information. In writing for practicing nurses, stress the application of material and concepts" (Sheridan & Dowdney, 1984).

This is not to say that editors want articles on any topic you indiscriminately select from your setting. Rather, select topics that provide new and innovative ideas for other practicing nurses. "Generate a clearcut idea with an original slant or point of view," said Helen Yura, coauthor of the book first describing nursing process (Sheridan & Dowdney, 1984). "Select a topic that is relevant, timely—with a different perspective than that presented in the literature . . . Don't presume anything! Have something to say! If you're going to spend the time, take time to do it well," said M. Janice Nelson, a director of nursing at a major New York medical center (Sheridan & Dowdney, 1984).

Writing about basics and fundamentals is another possibility because times and the field change. "When something in your own life changes—when, for example, you find yourself with an aging parent who can no longer live alone—you also inadvertently find yourself doing some research. What will you do? What kinds of resources are there? Is the problem of the elderly a problem with no solution? Will you have to think about a nursing home? . . . No writer can go through that kind of intense personal crisis without coming away with something significant to write. Granted, it's all been written before. But the problem of the elderly is evergreen—it'll be with us for a long, long time, and it renews itself every day as more people find themselves involved in the same situation" (Spikol, 1984, p. 14). In fact, the increasing numbers in our aging population, sometimes called "the greying of America," make this "old" topic current again.

Speeches and Lectures

Speeches that you present are other sources for article ideas. Sister Rosemary Donley perfected this process: "I usually give a speech and rework the ideas into a paper." Margaret L. McClure uses a similar approach. "Most of the articles that I have published in the past were oral presentations that I had given (Sheridan & Dowdney, 1984)." If you present classroom lectures or continuing education workshops, consider working these into articles.

Why not write up a lecture as an article? asked Donna Diers, when she was dean and professor at Yale School of Nursing.

> You already have the references, you have the feedback from the class about which points are the important ones and which ones bored them to sleep. . . . I am astonished by how infrequently faculty think of turning their lectures into articles or books. . . . Do you do in-service education? Do you speak to garden clubs or Rotary, or your church group or your jogging club about health or nursing, or something related? Do you write to your college roommate about the patient you've just cared for? Do you argue points of care over coffee with your colleagues? Do you go to professional organization meetings, prepare testimony for public hearings, debate with a doctor? Do you read articles in journals and criticize the foolish thinking of the author to your friends? Do you even sit around and brood about the state of nursing, or the state of the world, or the rottenness of your administrator, or the nastiness of the med students? Any occasion is grist for the writing mill . . . any firmly held conviction, any thoughtful critique, any vested emotional energy is a potential spark for the writing fire. (Diers, 1981, pp. 3–8)

Mary Maxwell (1981) wrote, "Scientific advances are communicated in preliminary form at professional meetings with the expectation that a complete article will follow in the literature" (p. 73). Even task forces and committees addressing particular needs or problems usually have article material from the results of the process.

Reading

Another source of ideas is reading what other nurses are writing in current journals. These may stimulate spin-off ideas. Donna Diers suggests, "Read a whole lot. Then write and write and write and write. Write about what you know and feel strongly about." She also said, "The best preparation for writing is reading. One learns to write, not only in formal settings and classrooms, but by reading the work of others and paying attention to the way words are used. Reading does not have to be confined to the esoteric, or the professional literature. Any piece composed of words is fair game for learning about writing. Obviously, the better the writing, the better the learning" (Diers, 1981, pp. 3–8).

When you disagree with something you read, challenge it. A healthy sign of a profession is members questioning each other. In a letter to the editor of *Image* (1994, p. 89), Kathleen B. King and Lisa H. Norsen question the "medical model, single cause, single cure" analogy as outdated, simplistic, and untrue, saying "When a pediatric nurse practitioner sees a child with a sore throat, makes a diagnosis, and writes a prescription, she's curing as well as caring." Their challenge of the care/cure, nurse/physician dichotomy is in response to an earlier article in *Image* on tertiary nurse practitioners. After applauding this article and much of its content, the authors raise their issues. Both the original article authors, and the authors of the letter to the editor are helping nursing to be a healthy profession by writing on opposing sides of a controversial topic. You can also raise questions with full-length scholarly articles of rebuttal.

Research

Research articles offer nurses a basis for practice. Your application of research may open publishing opportunities for you. Research journals are also a source of ideas for replicating studies or conducting new studies. Reading research may suggest ideas about articles to support or critique studies.

The format of the *Western Journal of Nursing Research* is especially helpful in suggesting further research and raising good questions. Through a forum format, commentaries by experts often follow the articles. These commentaries may be followed by a rebuttal from the authors if they desire to respond. Raising questions brings about ideas for you to pursue either through research or through writing an "opinion" type of article.

The most obvious source of ideas for research articles is the results of your own research. Try to frame your work problems into research questions and look for opportunities to pursue nursing research. Then, of course, your research should be shared through publication that can improve practice.

Journal Sections

Another source of writing ideas comes from looking at nursing journal sections. New nurse writers may want to try writing for a "department" of a journal such as "Speak Up" in *RN*; "Letters to the Editor" in most journals, or "Reflections" in *AJN*. These sections offer an opportunity to write a briefer article using a structured format. This may be particularly helpful if you have an idea that "just fits" one of these sections. Most journals have departments related to their themes. Look at these sections both as a place to target your articles, and as sources of ideas for expanded or refuted articles and themes to develop. *Nursing 96* has a number of departments to which new authors could submit articles.

- Confidentially—Brief anecdotes demonstrating important lessons nurses have learned from mistakes they've made (author's anonymity is guaranteed).
- Myths and Facts—A point-by-point debunking of prevalent misconceptions about different topics from diseases to various aspects of nursing care (see recent issue for format and sample topics).
- Sharing—One-page story describing dramatic, moving, or interesting personal experiences worth sharing with other nurses because of a valuable lesson learned.
- Self-Test—Challenging, multiple-choice questions on all aspects of nursing care, with answers at the end.
- Charting Tips—Prepares nurses to handle unusual charting challenges—and to avoid common documentation pitfalls.
- Combating Infection—Techniques, tips, and advice for preventing hospital-based infections.

See a current issue of the publication to determine which department would be the best for your article.

In *The Journal of Emergency Nursing,* (1984) Editor Gail Pisarcik Lenehan also suggested new authors begin by writing for sections:

> For Emergency Department nurses and other emergency healthcare providers who would like to write for *JEN* but aren't sure where to begin, a contribution to a section might be the answer—an Incidentally hint, a case review, or a news item for the Update section. Except for the legal column, every section welcomes contributions. . . . As for the Clinical Articles Section, we are particularly interested in publishing material such as current literature reviews; original research; content of interest to persons involved in various emergency nursing roles such as flight nurses, ED managers, clinical specialists, ED pediatric nurses and nurses working in emergency medical services systems; state-of-the-art of a facet of emergency nursing or emergency care; new programs; relevant regulatory news; exploration of issues affecting emergency nurses and emergency care; and articles that connote a positive, sophisticated image of emergency nursing. (pp. 1–2)

Besides emergency department specialty nurse writers, the editor indicated that *JEN* always needs to hear from experts in many different areas—nurses and others involved in infection control, trauma nursing, orthopedics, intensive care of neonates, pediatrics, infectious disease, cardiology, the medical/legal aspects of nursing, psychiatry and psychology, pharmacy, poison control centers, and countless other areas in which up-to-date information is necessary.

Another opportunity for "breaking in" is to publish first for a newsletter. These brief columns are "to the point" and usually "how-to" in nature. The number of newsletters are growing greatly as the pace and volume of information continue to accelerate. Newsletters quickly capture "the guts" of an article. These articles are not as in-depth as journal articles but provide a complement to the nursing literature. Examples include *Staff Development Insider* by Mosby Year Book and *Aspen's Advisor for Nurse Executives*, an Aspen Publication, or a local newsletter such as California's *Nurseweek*.

Television

Television can be another source for article ideas. Art Spikol, columnist for *Writer's Digest*, commented (1983):

> TV's main worth to a writer is its live interviews and news programs and, of course, its ability to show us the world. And any writer can tap in. For instance, if you see that Bill Buckley's "Firing Line" will be devoted to an interview which could either act as a springboard for a possible article or flesh out an article you're writing, you can tape the program and have what amounts to "live quotations" which won't usually appear elsewhere. Likewise, you could come across public television programming on dozens of subjects—interviews, films, specials—which could add to your knowledge on a particular subject. (p. 12)

Television programs often require nursing's response to reinforce or correct or challenge the content. Editorials need to be written to both nursing and nonnursing audiences in response to shows, explaining realities about health care education, disease prevention, health care system and practice realities, and nursing image portrayal.

There is also an opportunity to write for television. Donna Hill Howes, described as the "media mogul of the nursing profession" (Gray, 1995) encourages nurses to write, publish, and speak on healthcare. Howes, the only nonphysician on the Board of the Academy of Radio and Television Health Professionals, notes that consumers have an insatiable desire for healthcare information and don't want information just from physicians. Howes is expecting to have an ongoing nursing program on the new CNN 24-hour health channel—this should provide you with ideas to write on . . . and perhaps television opportunities also!

Radio and Newspapers

Talk shows on radio point out the most controversial topics of the moment that offer many ideas for development. Recently talk shows have addressed such topics as child abuse, hospital downsizing and closures, healthcare reform, school lunch nutrition, teen pregnancy, gangs, guns in the home, HIV, and sexuality. All of these subjects lend themselves to articles by nurses, the largest professional group in healthcare. The *New York Times,* the *Washington Post* and the *Los Angeles Times* conducted a 3-month survey determining sources for healthcare stories in their publications. Despite the profession's status in volume, and the fact that nurses have the most patient contact, nurses were the least quoted members of the healthcare professions. "Nurses do not see themselves as authority figures," says Howes. "It really has to start with us. We need to realize we are a valuable source of information" (Gray, 1995). During Nurse Week one year, Paul Harvey extolled the value of nurses on his radio show, "News and Comment." His statements were as powerful and effective as most nurses could present. With "nursing image" an ongoing concern in nursing, and thus a popular topic in the literature, Harvey's words offered a series of ideas for articles. Charles Osgood and Dan Rather also offer thought-producing topics that can lead to articles.

Ideas from Editors

You can request a list of upcoming topics or topics in which journal editors have an interest. You can also inquire about whether the publication follows particular themes. For example, *Nursing Administration Quarterly (NAQ)* focused its Winter 1995 issue on "gender issues in the workplace: breaking the glass ceiling." *Nursing & Health Care,* the official publication of the National League for Nursing (NLN) also uses themes. For example, their May 1993 issue focused on "Assuring the community's health." *NAQ* always follows themes—one per issue. Upcoming themes are printed on the backs of their issues or are available from the editor.

A new publication, *Nurse Author & Editor*™·, helps authors find a publisher interested in their work. It is a quarterly publication edited by Suzanne Hall Johnson, MN, RN, C, CNS (see "Foreword: A Nurse Editor's Perspective on page xi), which provides up-to-date information from nursing editors on topics they are looking for, and even on editorial board opportunities. Articles give advice to authors, editors, and editorial board members on writing, editing, and reviewing manuscripts for nursing articles or books. Also included is information on publishing inhouse nursing publications and writing for consumer magazines. *Nurse Author & Editor*™

is published by Hall Johnson Communications, 9737 West Ohio Ave., Lakewood, CO 80226. Contact them for subscription information.

Topics from Journal Editors

Editors would like to see articles on the following topics:

Alternative Health Practitioner: The Journal of Complementary and Natural Care
Meditation, guided imagery, therapeutic touch, acupressure, chiropractic, massage therapy, reflexology, rolfing, osteopathic medicine, nutrition and lifestyle change, art therapy, relaxation, biofeedback, hypnotherapy, acupuncture, herbs, homeopathy, and other related disciplines and procedures.

AORN Journal
Ambulatory surgery, lasers, management, and product evaluations.

Critical Care Nurse
Burns, trauma, neurosurgery, respiratory pathophysiology, gastrointestinal problems in the critically ill, and care of the critically ill surgical patient.

Health
Food, nutrition, beauty, psychology, fitness, kids, medical advances, and strongly angled medical stories.

Health Education
No parameters. Anything current, philosophical, or historical (in health).

Heart and Lung: Journal of Critical Care
New technical developments in critical care.

Hospitals
Almost all business aspects of the health care field.

Imprint
Nursing issues and no clinical papers.

Journal of Aging and Ethnicity
Aging among the diverse ethnic groups in North America. New immigrants from different countries and disparate cultures. Complexity of issues facing researchers, educators, policy and analysts, and practitioners in the field of aging. Research, education, policy, and practice related to aging among long-established and new immigrant populations.

Journal of Case Management
Case management philosophy and practice in private and institutional settings. Technology, law, business perspectives, insurance, third-party

financial affairs, computer technology, and reviews of literature and videos.

Examples of articles published in Volume 3, 1994 included

- Service utilization among older people with AIDS: Implications for case management
- Case management in Alzheimer's Disease
- Case management activities for the rural elderly: Findings from a national study

Journal of Emergency Nursing

Clinical topics. In particular, current state-of-the-art updates and reports of cases; also programs or projects that are new/innovative, and of course, relevant studies.

Journal of Ethics, Law, and Aging

Ethical and legal implications of the planning and administration of health care and social services for older persons and their families. Application of ethical principles and legal considerations for the practice of geriatrics and gerontology.

Journal of Long-Term Home Health Care

Research and analysis of current issues. Programs in long-term home health care. Special issues focused on Ethical Issues in Long Term Care; Homeless Elders: Prevention and Intervention; Alcohol Use and Abuse in the Aged; Cultural Competence in the Care of Elderly Chinese Persons; and Caring for the Difficult Patient at Home.

Examples of articles published in Volume 13, 1994, included

- Mechanisms of falls in community-residing older persons
- Recognizing and responding to elder maltreatment
- Youth exchanging With seniors: A rural Texas program
- Assessing the needs of persons of advanced age: The Weston, Massachusetts Council on Aging
- Continuing care retirement communities

Journal of Nurse-Midwifery

Clinical innovations relevant to nurse-midwifery.

Journal of Nursing Administration

Cost containment, computer applications in nursing, service and administration, corporate nursing, and nursing response to DRGs and Prospective Payment System (PPS).

Journal of Nursing Jocularity

Parodies and satires of nursing, medicine, and anything in a serious nursing or medical journal. Poems, song parodies, original games and puzzles, true stories about funny nursing experiences, information about therapeutic humor, articles or research about using humor and a positive attitude to relieve stress and promote wellness.

Journal of Nursing Measurement

Instruments, tools, approaches, and procedures developed or used to measure variables in nursing. Spans practice, education, and research. Examples of articles published in Volume 2, 1994 included

- Measurement of mealtime interactions among persons with dementing disorders
- A quantitative survey to measure energy expenditure in mid-life women
- Measurement of functional ability in patients with coronary artery disease

Journal of Obstetric, Gynecologic and Neonatal Nursing

Gynecology, oncology, wellness, contraceptives, sexually transmitted diseases, obstetrics, and neonatal nursing.

Nursing 96

Clinical articles describing particular diseases, disorders, or conditions, with the emphasis on relevant nursing care. Clinical articles focusing on specific assessment techniques, such as assessing heart sounds. Drug articles focusing on important nursing considerations related to preparing and administering drugs, potential adverse reactions, and careful evaluation of patient response. Charting/documentation articles that help nurses do this task more accurately and efficiently. Emotional problems that patients or their families encounter, such as anger or grief, and how nurses can help them cope. Legal problems nurses face in their daily work, such as floating, confidentiality, and informed consent. Ethical dilemmas nurses play a role in resolving; difficult or challenging cases that require good nursing skills. Teamwork. Resourcefulness.

Nursing Diagnosis

Nursing diagnosis.

Nursing Leadership Forum

Leadership with patients and families, nursing staff, health care institutions, or the larger community. Nursing leadership entering the public health care debate, setting future directions for the profession, and making an impact on the nation's health care. Exploration of values, ethics, and theories underlying nursing leadership.

Oncology Nursing Forum

Cancer nursing care and cancer treatment technology with nursing implications

Pediatric Nursing

Oncology, cardiac problems, chronic illness, eye infections, asthma, hematology, pain in infants, and research articles.

Scholarly Inquiry for Nursing Practice

Integration of theory, research, and practice. Quantitative and qualitative research, both basic and applied. State-of-the-art reviews and theory-based tool development. A renowned scholar's response accompanies each article. The scholar constructively examines the paper's relevance to practice.

Examples of topics in volume 8, 1994 included

- Nurse practitioner-patient discourse: Uncovering the voice of nursing in primary care practice
- Experienced and skilled nurses' narratives of situations where caring action made a difference to the patient
- Predictors of children's self-care performance: Testing the theory of self-care deficit

Today's OR Nurse

Surgical specialty procedures such as pediatrics, orthopedics, high technology equipment use, and education/orientation.

Personal Experience

Other idea sources for article topics may come from clinical, administrative, or educational experiences. To write the clinical article "119 Days in the ICU: Nursing Buster Back from the Brink," the authors looked no further than their everyday work setting. They wrote about a syndrome not new to the literature—Guillain-Barré. Yet the article is unique in the approach to the clinical and emotional challenges they faced in this "case study" type of article. The authors described the disease progression through a framework of sequential feelings—love, empathy, inadequacy, optimism, exasperation, guilt, inspiration, frustration, anger, and gratification. A sidebar (inset) in the article briefly refreshed readers on the signs, symptoms, clinical course, and treatment of Guillain-Barré without rewriting about an already known subject (Anderson et al., 1985).

Another topic, clinical ladders, again not new to the literature, was well addressed in an article entitled "Implementing a Clinically Focused Advancement System: One Institution's Experience" (Hamric, Whitworth, Greenfield, 1993). Sharing a program from their own institution with the profession, these authors updated the nursing literature with their personal experience and allowed others to learn how to update the time-tested ladders, while avoiding the pitfalls that have historically caused ladders to fail.

In education, as in clinical and administrative settings, article topics are readily available. For example, as Indiana University's School of Nursing prepared for its 1990 National League for Nursing (NLN) accreditation under the auspices of a "system" school, their self evaluation and preparation was intense. In an article "Self-Evaluation in a Complex System-Wide School of Nursing" (Adams & McBride, 1993) two professors shared their comprehensive plan, noting specifically their eight major success strategies. Although the authors didn't need to look for this personal experience, their efforts, now shared in the literature, offer guidance to other nursing schools nationally.

And in their everyday work setting in Evanston, Illinois, nurses learned about and wrote about "Guillain-Barré Syndrome: Giving the Patient Control" (Anderson, 1992)—still timely and still useful in the literature.

Nurse educators now have a whole new world of publishing opportunities by writing for the "Earn CEU" type of articles that many journals carry. Even a common topic such as congestive heart failure can be worked into a continuing education article, as Kathleen McCauley did in "Congestive Heart Failure: A Step by Step Guide to Better Nursing Management" (1984). This can also be done for nonclinical topics. The *Journal of Nursing Administration* published "Procedure Development: A Simplified Approach" (Griffith & Ignatavicius, 1984).

Problem-Solving Situations

Problem-solving situations often make excellent article topics. In "Self-Scheduling: A Strategy for Recruitment and Retention" (Tully, 1992) authors deal with schedule-related low morale and conflict between staff members by implementing self-scheduling. Not a new concept, but still effective; these authors share the tools and process of their problem-solving with "how-tos" related to planning, pitfalls with suggestions of what to avoid, guidelines for scheduling, and outcomes of their project.

Keeping a complete and accurate physical assessment record of spinal cord injury patients is a problem Laura Caramanica solved by using an assessment flowsheet at Yale New Haven Hospital. She shared her useful tool in an article published by *Dimensions of Critical Care Nursing (DCCN)* (Caramanica, 1984).

Relationships with Others

Some editors will also welcome articles about ways to improve relationships with co-workers. If you have enhanced a team spirit between nurses and physicians or nurses and administrators, or if you have enhanced the nursing image or promoted professionalism, why not share that success in an article? In "Conflict and Retention of New Graduate Nurses", (Gardner, 1992) the author examines the types of conflicts perceived by graduate nurses in their first year of work. Job conflict was found to be inversely related to job satisfaction, which may be linked to retention. The article's concepts are applicable to many relationships in conflict, including those resulting from the presence of more seasoned nurses in a changing organization.

Nonnursing Issues

Another source of ideas comes from nonnursing experiences or significant environmental changes to nursing. How is nursing affected by what is happening in the world? Why should nurses become more involved in legal, environmental, or political nonnursing issues? You might consider developing a letter to send to an editor of a professional publication on a nonnursing topic you would like to air. Include its impact or potential impact on nursing. Jennifer Lillard wrote a thought-provoking letter to the editor of *Oncology Nursing Forum* (1984) dealing with nuclear responsibility. She linked her involvement in hospice nursing with issues concerning nuclear war.

Basic Human Needs

Additional sources of writing ideas come from basic human needs such as food, shelter, clothing, finding and keeping a mate, sexual desire and gratification, pregnancy and childrearing, family relationships, companionship, avoiding danger, and preserving health. For example, Skoner, Thompson, and Caron (1994) investigated and wrote on "Factors Associated with Risk of Stress Urinary Incontinence in Women." Sports, hobbies, vacations, travel, and recreation are other possibilities for showing how nursing activities can improve health.

For example, decreasing anxiety in the myocardial infarction patient through music therapy was explored by nurses at Marquette University College of Nursing (White, 1992). Similarly, in Hunstville, Alabama, nurses explored the effects of ocean sounds on sleep after coronary artery bypass surgery knowing that deprivation of sleep can impede repair. In fact, patients listening to ocean waves slept more deeply and woke less frequently during the night. Perhaps the nurse designing this study and article had just returned from a cruise.

LIST IDEAS

After you consider the many potential manuscript ideas surrounding you, take several minutes to list ideas you might be able to develop into journal articles. Do not reject any idea because it seems too complicated, too unconventional, or too mundane. Write down even outrageous ideas without judging them.

James Adams, author of *Conceptual Blockbusting,* wrote

> If you analyze or judge too early . . . you will reject many ideas. This is detrimental for two reasons. First of all, newly formed ideas are fragile and imperfect—they need time to mature and acquire the detail needed to make them believable. . . . Second, ideas often lead to other ideas. Many techniques of conceptualization, such as brainstorming, depend for their effectiveness on maintaining "way-out" ideas long enough to let them mature and spawn other more realistic ideas. It is sometimes difficult to hold to such ideas because people generally do not want to be suspected of harboring impractical thoughts. However, in conceptualization one should not judge too quickly (1974, pp. 46–47).

BRAINSTORMING

The well-known technique of brainstorming is a group problem-solving method useful in generating topic ideas. Through the technique of brainstorming, an environment conducive to creativity is artificially set up to stimulate and protect large quantities of "sudden inspirations" by agreeing to ground rules:

- Think of the wildest ideas possible.
- Strive for quantity of ideas because quantity will lead to quality.
- Do not criticize or judge any ideas because group members will become more concerned with defending ideas than with generating them.
- Build new ideas on ideas already suggested.

This technique is usually used in a group. You can use it that way with a coauthor, a nurse writers' group, a task force, a committee, or at a staff meeting of nurses wanting to write a group article or stimulate ideas for individual articles. You can also use the technique as an individual.

Remember, in brainstorming, quantity, not quality, is important. Think of and write down as many ideas as quickly as you can. Often one idea provokes another or a new idea comes from a combination of some earlier ideas. Don't judge any ideas; the more outrageous, the better. When you think you are out of ideas, keep on thinking and writing. Often the best ideas emerge after you think you have no more ideas.

Some people brainstorm as a first writing step, before deciding about purpose and audience needs, just to get started. Others brainstorm only after writing a rough draft. Regardless of the sequence, good writers usually brainstorm at some stage in the process, to ensure they discover *all* the material readers might find useful. (Lannon, 1994, p. 28)

Ask questions to enhance your list, using "who, what, when, where, why, and how" to help you review your current setting and come up with more ideas. For example, "Who did I care for this week? What was unique about the care? What is my next educational program topic? How have we cut costs and maintained quality?"

You can generate a list of questions related to nursing in general or your work setting. Then generate a list of answers to each. Your ideas will begin to fill pages. When you are finished listing the ideas, look for modifications or new combinations to see if they offer additional possibilities. Be as imaginative as possible. Generate additional ideas by considering new viewpoints. For example, if you are writing about unique nursing needs of postpartum patients over 40, ask yourself, Who are these patients? What are their needs? When do they have these needs? How can you meet these needs? and so forth.

Examine a variety of nursing journals to increase your idea list. Do not write the same ideas, but use the current articles to spark your own ideas. Especially review letters to the editor for "coming" topics and issues.

SELECT A TOPIC

From your idea list, select one topic to develop into a journal article. Some factors to consider in choosing your topic are your personal interest in the subject and how current the topic is in nursing publications. It is unlikely you will complete an article if you do not find the topic interesting before you begin writing. The subject must interest you enough to carry you through the process of investigating and reading about it, then writing and editing.

Editors do not want stale articles. If most nurses already know about your topic, editors probably will not be interested unless you have new information. To determine if a topic involves generally known facts, look at current nursing textbooks. If the topic already appears in a textbook, the information is old. If you are writing on an old topic, be sure to write from a new perspective.

To be current, review the periodical literature. Finding your topic in current literature is a positive sign. You may think the opposite—"Someone has already written my manuscript." On the contrary, many approaches to a topic are possible. Not only is a variety of viewpoints essential for the profession, but a unique slant to a timely topic is a desirable addition to nursing literature.

For example, when Diagnosis Related Groups (DRGs) became a reimbursement issue for hospitals, and thus for nursing, the literature became saturated with DRG articles. In 1983, "Diagnosis Related Groups" was not even a heading in the *Cumulative Index to Nursing and Allied Health Literature* (1983). Any related topics were listed under "Insurance," "Health," or "Reimbursement." In 1984, only one year later, the Index listed almost two pages of references to DRG articles—over 120 articles. Some titles included: "What's DRG's Impact on Home Health?" (Zimmerman-Cathcart, 1983); "DRGs: de revenue's gone . . . a Unique Opportunity for Nurses" (Mitchell, 1984); and "DRGs and RIMs: Implications for Nursing" (Joel, 1984). General nursing journals, specialty journals, management journals, and educational journals all carried articles on this hot issue, each slanted to an individual journal market. A variety of viewpoints on this hot topic was essential because of this legislation's impact on health care institutions and nursing practice. Those authors whose articles were published gave their articles a slant unique to the journal in which they published. Today, DRGs are not as hot. In 1994 only five articles are referenced on DRGs in the *Cumulative Index to Nursing & Allied Health Literature* (CINAHL)—two of these are about DRGs in Australia, and two are about DRGs in pediatrics.

An example of a clinical "hot issue" that surfaced swiftly in the literature was Acquired Immunodeficiency Syndrome (AIDS) in response to the many questions being raised in the nursing profession due to major increase in incidence. Authors who were quick to react to the questions and knew or found out about the best answers available at the time wrote and had their manuscripts published.

For example, Jerold Cohen (1984) wrote "AIDS," a brief (less than 1,000 words) explanatory article including only an introduction, nursing implications, and a summary. Two of the three references he cited were from the Centers for Disease Control (CDC), and the other was "Facts about AIDS" published by the U.S. Department of Health and Human Services. This author was among the first to write on a timely topic, finding good sources of information and an interested audience. "AIDS—Safety Practices for Clinical and Research Laboratories" was written for a very different audience and published in *Infection Control* (Federico & Gershon, 1984). A less technical treatment of the topic was carried by *Nursing 83*, "Caring for the AIDS Patient—Fearlessly" (Popkin, 1983). Ten years later, dozens of articles continue in the literature addressing the topic of AIDS. In addition, several journals have developed dedicated to this topic including: *AIDS Alert, AIDS Education Prevention,* and *AIDS Patient Care,* all indexed in CINAHL.

After thorough treatment of hot issues in the literature, the journal acquisition editors do not want to see the topics again unless what you have to say is very different and important to their readers. However, while the issue is still unresolved or incidence continues to climb, new slants to the topic are still possible.

When selecting your topic, consider whether it involves a recurring theme in nursing. Some topics in nursing never leave the literature. Better approaches are continually sought. Gordon Burgett (1980), author of over 900 articles, said, "Some general topics are evergreens, always in bloom and always in print." Then he listed the following "evergreens": "New ways of doing old things, better ways to use resources, ways to spark self-motivation, family involvement with patients, more effective policies and procedures, and methods of keeping professionally fresh and involved" (p. 43).

"Dealing with the Angry Employee" (Dorman, 1984) is not a new topic. A 1990's version may look more like "The Executive's Role in Getting Everyone Aboard: Coping with Individual Response to Collective Change" (Kane, 1992). This article explores how understanding the behaviors of recalcitrant individuals can guide interventions for positive outcomes. Continually timely topics include: "Managing Effective Meetings" (Jacobs & Rosenthal, 1984) and "Ten Criteria for Effective Team Building" (Kazemek, 1991), both useful as long as we continue to spend large amounts of time in these activities. And "Bedside Assessment of the Myocardial Infarction Patient" is not a new clinical topic. Assessment articles are continually useful to resurface periodically in the literature, perhaps with an update or new slant. In *AJN* Stiesmeyer offers for continuing education credit "A Four Step Approach to Pulmonary Assessment" (1993).

The fast pace of the changing economy, technology, and health care creates some article ideas not seen in past nursing literature. For instance, "An Approach to Funding Nursing Continuing Education Conferences" (Hopkin & Perlich, 1985); "Comparable Worth: Alternatives to Litigation and Legislation" (Youngkin, 1985); and "Hybridoma Monoclonal Antibody Treatment of T-Cell Lymphomas: Clinical Experience and Nursing Management" (Di Julio & Bedigian, 1983) were not issues until the last decade. And now you may need to read up on topics in the literature on Carpal Tunnel Syndrome, Help-Seeking Behaviors, Verapamil, or Multiskilled Health Practitioners.

Consider whether you want to write on a topic that interests a specialized group of nurses, or whether you want to write a more general article that would evoke wide interest in the nursing community. Sometimes you might develop the same topic either way. For example, the subject of contact lenses was covered by two journals with very different treatments. The

Journal of Gerontological Nursing (Hall, 1984) published an article entitled, "Extended Wear Contact Lenses: What Nurses Should Know." The article explained that the aphakic elder client needs nursing help to care for and note complications in extended wear lenses. Another article, "The Ins and Outs of Contact Lenses" (Carden, 1983) focused on how nurses can help hospitalized contact lens wearers when their tolerance for wearing their lenses is affected by illness, drugs, and changed sleeping patters. These articles are similar, but are developed in different ways, one to appeal to a general nursing readership and the other for readers in the specialized gerontology field. Today's nurse still needs to know this information about contact lenses, and articles continue to be published on the topic, with slanting toward scleral lenses or lense-related bacterial infections. A journal even exists for nurses in this specialty, *The Journal of Ophthalmic Nursing Technology.*

When choosing which topic to write on, consider all of the following:

- How well do you know the topic?
- Are you interested in the topic?
- Does it fall within your area of expertise?
- Do you have access to enough data to write a quality article?
- Will the topic be of interest to other nurses?
- Is the scope feasible?
- Are there any ethical considerations?
- Can you share the information?
- Should you involve others in collaboration?
- Is it part of a grant request—and what are the grant stipulations?
- Will publication on this topic enhance your professional growth and opportunities?
- Is it a field in which you would like to become known?
- Would you want to consult or speak in this field?

As you think about publishing what you practice, choose topics that are important to you—topics about which you feel a strong, even passionate interest. If you choose a topic you feel is vital, exciting, and important, you will feel satisfied when it is published that you have communicated your ideas to others.

After considering possible topics in light of your expertise, interest in the subject, and other criteria mentioned above, select one topic to work on now. If you have more than one favorite topic, choose the one that holds the greatest appeal for you. That one will be the easiest to complete. Perhaps you have performed research or presented a speech in this area. Whatever topic you select, stick with it through this book. Use each step of the writing process to develop that idea into a journal article.

Save your topic list for future article ideas. Whenever you think of a new topic or idea, add it to this list. Now is a good time to set up information files. In these files, tape or staple the topic idea list to a large envelope or manila folder. Place references, related articles, and bibliographical information inside the files as you come across it. As you discover other topics, continue to add them to your list.

EXERCISE

Brainstorm a list of possible topics for journal articles. For several days add to that list as you generate more ideas using the following sources:

- Patient care experiences
- Problems you have solved
- Opinions about nursing education or image
- Legislative and economic changes
- Committee and project work
- Information systems
- Journal themes
- Nursing journal articles
- Nursing journal indices
- Nursing journal sections
- Workshops and classes
- Current nonnursing topics you could relate to nursing in education, pharmacology, management, finance, physiology, economics, sociology, etc.
- Technological changes
- Television and radio

REFERENCES

Adams, C. J., & McBride, A. B. (1993). Self evaluation in a complex system-wide school of nursing. *Nursing & Health Care, 14,* 462–464.

Adams, J. L. (1974). *Conceptual blockbusting.* New York: W. W. Norton.

Anderson, B. S. (1992). Guillain-Barré syndrome: Giving the patient control. *Journal of Neuroscience Nursing, 24,* 158–162.

Anderson, D., Null, J., Miller, B., Tornabeni, J., O'Brien, B., & Platt, J. (1985, January). 119 days in the ICU: Nursing Buster back from the brink. *RN. 48*(1), 30–36.

Burgett, G. L. (1980, November-December). Writing an article for a nursing journal. *The Journal of Practical Nursing, 30,* 43.

Caramanica, L. (1984). Assessment flowsheet for spinal cord injury. *Dimensions of Critical Care Nursing, 3*(3), 147–153.

Carden, R. G. (1985, February). The ins and outs of contact lenses. *RN, 48*(2), 48–50.

Cohen, J. (1984). AIDS. *Imprint, 13*(4), 50.

Cumulative index to nursing and allied health literature [CINAHL]. (1984). *29*(6).

Diers, D. (1981). Why write? Why publish? *Image, 13*(5), 3–8.

Di Julio, J. E., & Bedigian, J. S. (1983). Hybridoma monoclonal antibody treatment of T-cell lymphomas: Clinical experience and nursing management. *Oncology Nursing Forum, 10*(2), 22–27.

Dorman, D. D. (1984). Dealing with the angry employee. *Health Care Supervisor Today, 2*(4), 13–23.

Dowdney, D. L., & Sheridan, D. R. (1984). *Survey of nursing and health care journal editors.* Unpublished manuscript.

Federico, J. V., & Gershon, R. R. M. (1984). AIDS—Safety practices for clinical and research laboratories. *Infection Control, 5*(4), 185–187.

French, D. G. (1984, November). Ethics: Nurse am I going to live? *Nursing Management, 15*(11), 43–46.

Gardner, D. L. (1992). Conflict and retention of new graduate nurses. *Western Journal of Nursing Research, 14*(1), 76–85.

Gray, B. (1995). RN says nurses must get involved in media. *Nurseweek, 8*(3), 1, 20.

Griffith, J., & Ignatavicius, D. (1984). Procedure development: A simplified approach. *Journal of Nursing Administration, 14*(9), 27–32.

Hall S. S. (1984). Extended-wear contact lenses: What nurses should know. *Journal of Gerontological Nursing, 10*(6), 28, 29, 33.

Hamric, A. B., Whitworth, T. R., & Greenfield, A. S. (1993). Implementing a clinically focused advancement system: One institution's experience. *Journal of Nursing Administration, 23*(9), 20–28.

Holtzclaw, B. J., Boggs, K. U., & Wilson, M. E. (1993). *Computers in Nursing, 11*(5), 242–248.

Hopkin, L. A. S., & Perlich, L. J. M. (1985). An approach to funding nursing continuing education conferences. *Nursing Economics, 3*(1), 33–37.

Jacobs, B. C., & Rosenthal, T. T. (1984). Managing effective meetings. *Nursing Economics, 2*(2), 137–141.

Joel, L. A. (1984). DRGs and RIMs: Implications for nursing. *Nursing Outlook, 32*(1), 42–49.

Kane, J. (1992). The executive's role in getting everyone aboard: coping with individual response to collective change. *Aspen's Advisor, 7*(1), 1–5.

Kazemek, E. A. (1991). Ten criteria for effective team building. *Healthcare Financial Management, 45,* 15.

King, K. B., & Norsen, L. H. (1994). The care/cure, nurse/physician dichotomy doesn't do it anymore [Letter to the editor]. *Image, Journal of Nursing Scholarship, 26*(2), 89.

Lannon, J. M. (1994). *Technical writing.* New York: Harpercollins College Publishers.

Lenehan, G. P. (1984). JEN looks in the mirror. *Journal of Emergency Nursing, 10*(1), 1–2.

Lillard, J. (1984). Nuclear responsibility. [Letter to the editor]. *Oncology Nursing Forum, 11*(2), 18.

Maxwell, M. B. (1981). Published or perished: What becomes of papers presented at Oncology Nursing Society Congresses? *Oncology Nursing Forum, 8*(3), 73.

McCauley, K. M. (1984). Congestive heart failure: A step by step guide to better nursing management. *Nursing Life, 4*(3), 33–40.

Mitchell, K. (1984). DRGs: De revenue's gone . . . a unique opportunity for nurses. (Editorial.) *Pediatric Nursing, 10*(5), 317.

Nursing 96 (1996). Writer's guidelines for *Nursing 96*. [On-line]. Available E-Mail: http://www.springnet.com/jrdescr/jrn-d41.htm#Style

Popkin, B. Madden, P., Lavich, P., & Sherlock, M. E. (1983, September). Caring for the AIDS patient—fearlessly. *Nursing, 13*(9), 50.

Schoenbaum, M. (1995). Recognizing Torsade de Pointes. *American Journal of Nursing, 95*(2), 54.

Sheridan, D. R., & Dowdney, D. L. (1984). *Survey of selected nurse authors.* Unpublished work.

Skoner, M. M., Thompson, W. D., & Caron, V. A. (1994). Factors associated with risk of stress urinary incontinence in women. *Nursing Research, 43,* 301–306.

Spikol, A. (1983, March). Ideas on ideas. *Writer's Digest,* 12.

Spikol, A. (1984, August). Colleague's complaint. *Writer's Digest,* 14.

Stiesmeyer, J. K. (1993). A four-step approach to pulmonary assessment. *American Journal of Nursing, 93*(8), 22–28.

Tully, K. C. (1992). Self scheduling: a strategy for recruitment and retention. *Focus on Critical Care, 19*(1), 69–73.

White, J. M. (1992). Music therapy: An intervention to reduce anxiety in the myocardial infarction patient. *Clinical Nurse Specialist, 6*(1), 58–63.

Youngkin, E. Q. (1985). Comparable worth: Alternatives to litigation and legislation. *Nursing Economics, 3*(1), 38–43.

Zimmerman-Cathcart, B. (1983). What's DRG's impact on home health? *Pennsylvania Nurse, 38*(10), 6, 8.

3

Develop a Plan

Developing your selected ideas into an article requires a plan. All well-written, published nursing articles begin with plans. Although all experienced nurse authors may not need to put their plans into writing, new writers will find that writing the plan clarifies thinking, identifies gaps, and focuses the manuscript. This chapter will help you develop your idea into a writing plan and will address some issues on beginning to focus your manuscript.

COLLABORATION

The first step in a writing plan is to decide whether you want to do your project alone or in collaboration with others. Collaboration, or teamwork, is an increasingly common approach to writing. More than one expert may need to solve a problem or develop products or systems. All or some of the same experts may then want to be involved in writing subsequent related articles. Similarly, articles may result from a committee or task force. The reward of publication may be important to all contributors—either as co-authors or as contributors. In some organizations, it could be advantageous to collaborate with the leader in the field. In other situations, one author may have writing and editing skills while the other may have the clinical and technical expertise. This writing team may be able to produce a stronger manuscript than either individual could alone.

Some of the advantages of collaboration include the synergistic effect of complementary skills, broader expertise, and sanction to share organizational projects in the literature.

Collaborating with another writer can more than double writing creativity, productivity, and energy. . . . Your collaborator doesn't even have to be another writer. A doctor or scientist working on a new diet theory or a cure for the common cold, for example, would presumably like to get his or her discoveries in front of the public. What's more, professionals of this sort can steer you to their clients or colleagues for interviews, thus saving you the time you would have spent scouting subjects on your own (Watson-Rouslin & Peck, 1985, pp. 32–34).

The problems, however, may outnumber the advantages. Many problems prevent potentially excellent articles from getting to press. This is not to say that you should avoid collaboration; rather, if you collaborate, you need to be aware of predictable areas of conflict. Decide early who will be the first author; do not wait until the title page is about to be typed for the final version. No failure in scholarly procedure is more likely to breed ill-will and wreck friendships and collegial relations than putting off decisions about authorship to a time when failure to agree may bring unpleasant consequences and even damage careers (Huth, 1982).

Difficulties surrounding the collaborative experience may arise

because most writing teams begin by attacking tasks without first completing some necessary preparatory steps. Teams function best when they first build the interpersonal environment necessary for their creative problem solving, consider possible approaches toward collaborating, decide on the ways they might handle conflict, access computer technologies to facilitate their work, and identify the strengths of their diverse members. Teams that generate a common understanding concerning their collaborative relationships and the process they will follow to complete their tasks are those that succeed. (Lay, et al., 1995)

Randomly selected nurse authors who had collaborated on journal articles responded candidly to our survey question dealing with collaboration (Sheridan & Dowdney, 1984). Their comments addressed their writing processes, decisions about designating first author, advantages and disadvantages of teamwork in writing, and their preferences for single or multiple authorship.

Most co-authors agreed that understandings must be reached early in the process: "We make our expectations clear at the beginning," said one nurse author. Another elaborated, "We set ground rules first to determine who is the best with which aspects of the work. We explore the audience, the focus of the article, and the content. Then we each take a portion of responsibility, depending on individual interest and areas of expertise.

We share written information and critique and alter drafts as we go" (Sheridan & Dowdney, 1984).

How the work is divided varies:

- "I do the outline and research, then I assign the portions of the outline."
- "I was responsible for the conceptualization and first draft. My second author contributed to the results section."
- "We draft an outline together. Then the drafts are written by a single author and passed back and forth for rewrites."
- "The first author usually reviews the literature and writes the methods. I often do the analysis and write the results. We do the discussion together."
- "I was the primary author; she simply reviewed it."
- "We had a 50/50 split in outlining the article, dividing the work, and assembling the article."
- "We divided according to each author's expertise."

Although the way in which authors divide their work varies, the important point is not how it is divided, but that it is agreed upon ahead and that all parties agree to the split. Sometimes, collaboration does not work out well—especially if work expectations are not clearly defined ahead. One nurse author said, "I did all the work." Another said, "I wrote it—she changed it—we forgot it!"

Who will be first author and the ordering of subsequent names is an important issue that needs to be addressed before any writing is done. Often this is a major factor in dividing the work. We asked nurse authors how they decide who will be the first author. Several responded that they used alphabetical order. More often it related to other factors:

- "The first author is the one who does the major writing or who has been funded by grant funds."
- "The first author is the writer who produces the first draft."
- "The first author is the one who had the idea for the article."
- "The first author is the one with the highest degree."
- "It is difficult. I gave in and let her be the first author."
- "We decide based on the amount of work involved and the publishing experience."
- "When it is the boss, position decides."
- "50/50. We take turns assuming first authorship."
- "We tossed a coin" (Sheridan & Dowdney, 1984).

Many nurse authors agree that collaboration has advantages. They said:

- "It provides encouragement, clarification of ideas, critique, and helps in setting deadlines."
- "It gives different points of view and more input."
- "It uses the strengths of different people."
- "It helps to have someone to talk to when you get tired of the subject."
- "It's fun, there's better depth, more ideas, and more publications."
- "It is less work for each person. Others also help to sustain motivation" (Sheridan & Dowdney, 1984).

However, collaboration is not without disadvantages. Different points of view, for example, may be seen as both an advantage and a disadvantage of collaboration. One nurse author believed that single or multiple authorship is not an issue. "There is no difference as long as it gets published," she wrote. Nurse authors commented that working with a co-author actually takes longer than single authorship because it is difficult to schedule sessions, and that co-authors slowed them down when they failed to meet deadlines, do their part, and share the workload. Some other disadvantages noted include:

- "You don't know when they will complete their revisions. Sometimes I have difficulty in getting the other author to do any work. It seems to take more time, which is the biggest disadvantage."
- "Style and deadlines vary."
- "Dividing up work, deciding order of authorship, and putting the sections of each author together so it flowed and language was consistent are problems."
- "Disagreements about style and philosophy could ruin friendships."
- "It's hard to collaborate from across the country."
- "Compromising on issues is a disadvantage" (Sheridan & Dowdney, 1984).

When we asked nurse authors whether they preferred single or multiple authorship, most chose single authorship and indicated the following reasons:

- "I work at a very organized and rapid pace, and many do not."
- "It is difficult to agree."
- "I do the work, and I want the credit."
- "You have more control over the material and writing style."
- "It takes less time, and I maintain control over the article. However, I

do have others read my articles and welcome feedback (Sheridan & Dowdney, 1984).

Some writers expressed preference for single or multiple authorship depending on the article content, nature of the work, and other current responsibilities and time demands:

- "There are pros and cons to both. As a single author, you have total control of all aspects: content, style, and pace. However, it is also easy to know the information so well that the obvious may be omitted from the article."
- "I now include junior colleagues as first or second author for their professional development."
- "It depends on the subject matter and whether the work addressed in the article was independent or based on joint work and interest" (Sheridan & Dowdney, 1984).

In research, it is important to establish at the beginning of the research whether publications will result from the investigation—and an important part of research is the publication of the findings. This is also the time to agree upon co-authorship and the roles of co-authors in preparing research reports.

Frank E. McLaughlin (1981) wrote, "Oral agreements tend to be forgotten or misinterpreted during the life of the research project, thus written agreements are necessary. Attention to this crucial detail will prevent misunderstanding, frustration, or ill will later" (p. 38).

If you decide to write with one co-author or as part of a group, set up some ground rules and timeframes before you begin. Also determine the order of authors' names. On deciding who will do what, you may decide to each take specific parts of the writing process. The Writing Plan that follows will help you focus your article.

If you are a novice writer, you may have a better chance of seeing your article published if you have a coach or a friend to stimulate continued commitment and motivation. It might be especially helpful to work with a well-published author to learn about writing as you work together. However, do not hesitate to write alone if you think you work better this way. Just be sure to set and stick to deadlines and seek peer input.

Before you enter into a collaborative relationship, ask yourself the following key questions:

1. Will the collaborator's ideas or experience be of interest to a journal?
2. Does the collaborator have enough facts, theories, statistics, research, anecdotes, or case studies to draw upon for the article?

3. Will the collaborator give the project the time it requires?
4. Is the collaborator knowledgeable about what the writing process involves?

Using Computers to Collaborate

You may decide to collaborate on your writing projects with colleagues in distant locations by using electronic mail (e-mail) or local area networks (LANs). Computers allow you to plan, write, review, revise, edit, and read manuscripts online. When co-authors connect to a computer network, software allows you to merge the various parts of manuscripts. As you collaborate on your manuscripts using networking techniques, you use most of the traditional writing methods we describe in this book, but you will also develop some new work patterns. Herbert B. Michaelson (1990) described the following three ways to collaborate in network-based writing:

1. Various portions of the writing are prepared simultaneously by co-authors and then transmitted on the network to the senior author for combination into a completed manuscript. This is a horizontal division of the writing process.
2. Or, one person prepared a complete draft of the manuscript, which is then sent on the network to groups or individuals who successively edit the artwork and text, design the page layouts, and print the final report. Here, the collaboration is hierarchical.
3. Or, authors connected to the network share access to databases, using hypertext techniques of composition, and later combine their portions into a coherent manuscript. (pp. 171–172)

Nursing faculty in academic settings can communicate with colleagues nationally and internationally through electronic networks. Members of the Southern Nursing Research Society's Governing Board use electronic communication methods to accomplish the organization's work.

Chapter Five of this book includes information about performing online computer searches and using the Internet and online services. Tables include contact information for selected online services and software, selected online medical and health resources on CompuServe, forums on CompuServe of interest to nurses, and selected computer-readable databases of interest to nurses.

THE WRITING PLAN

In addition to making decisions about single or multiple authorship and, with the latter, division of work and name order, you also need to make several other significant decisions before you begin writing. Record decisions you make on the Writing Plan. You will be making decisions about your organizing idea, manuscript's purpose, organizing framework, working title, theme, theme development method, target audience, target journal, and time schedule. The Plan has three major components—the writing component, the marketing component, and the timeline.

Because the nature of the Writing Process is cyclical, do not worry about developing a perfect plan at this time. You will be refining the Plan as you use the process. Place a response on each line of the Plan as you read each segment below. The Writing Plan details the Writing Process presented in this book. The Plan will be easier to complete as you read upcoming chapters. Complete a Writing Plan (Figure 3.1) for each article you write.

The Idea

Select one idea from the list of ideas you generated in Chapter 2. If you selected more than one idea to develop, choose one to write on first. Stay with this idea throughout the book to learn the Writing Process. Because switching ideas is a symptom of writer's block, do not allow yourself to change ideas after you have selected one.

In the writing workshops we conduct, we ask for a commitment from all participants at the beginning of the workshop to stay with their chosen idea. Workshop participants have often been surprised that they could work through their writing blocks and have been glad they stayed with one idea to learn the Process. Often when writers become blocked, they blame the idea and select another. Therefore, select your idea carefully; then see it through to at least the query letter stage.

If you are a first-time writer, limit yourself to one idea while you learn the Process. After you become more skilled, you may find that working with more than one idea simultaneously makes good use of your time, particularly as you work in the library.

The Purpose of Your Manuscript

What do you want to say about your topic? What is your purpose for writing this manuscript? Why would another nurse want to read it? What do you want your reader to do or think? Some purposes for manuscripts are described below, with examples of each.

Are you writing to inform others by explaining facts? A popular theme for clinical nursing journals is nursing care related to new technological or medical developments. Some examples of informational articles are: "Neurotoxins: A Neuroscience Nursing Challenge" in the *Journal of Neuroscience Nursing* (Hinkle, 1994).

You may be writing to show others how to do something. "How-to" articles provide step-by-step instructions so that others can duplicate a process or procedure. Some examples are: "How to Stay Cool in a Conflict and Turn it into Cooperation" (Guttenberg, 1983); and "A Nurse's Guide to Tube Feeding" (Miller & Miller, 1995).

Are you writing to share a personal experience about an ordeal, process, or event? Personal experience articles inspire, educate, or entertain readers. "Writing from your own experience enables you to speak authoritatively, tap an extensive store of knowledge, attend to details, and develop your paper in a logical and meaningful manner" (O'Connor, 1980, pp. 22–23).

In "Going the Distance with the Patient Who's a Real Fighter" (Beaudoin, 1983), a team of nurses who committed themselves to helping a patient pull through a bone marrow transplant for leukemia shared some hard-learned lessons. A very different experience is shared in "Sheila Barnes Had a Knack for Making Me Feel Awkward" (Stein, 1983). The article stated, "This new grad had to deal with a difficult person right from the start. Intimidated by an older RN, she learned how to cope" (p. 1).

Sharing research results with your colleagues may be your purpose for writing. Some examples of articles written for this purpose include: "Mothers' Intention, Age, Education and the Duration and Management of Breastfeeding" published in *Maternal-Child Nursing Journal* (Quarles et al., 1994); and "A Study of Yoga as a Nursing Intervention in the Care of Patients with Pleural Effusion" (Prakasamma, 1984).

Besides sharing research studies, you may wish to show how to apply research to practice—"Understanding the Use of Basic Statistics in Nursing Research" (Weiner & Weiner, 1983); discuss human subjects' rights in research—"Protecting Children's Rights during Research" (Mitchell, 1984); and discuss nursing participation in research—"Should Critical Care Nurses Participate in Pharmacologic Research?" (Miller, 1984).

Inspiring others by showing successful efforts of individuals or groups learning to understand and improve a situation is another purpose you may have for writing. Examples include: "Reaching the Migrant Worker" (O'Brien, 1983); from a different perspective, "Collective Bargaining: Serving the Common Good in a Crisis" (Sargis, 1985); or even "Sally Had a Drug Habit but I Looked the Other Way" (Costello, 1984).

Your purpose might be to show a person's or organization's rise to success. On a personal level, Doreen Casey, a registered nurse, shares her freedom from the grip of drugs and alcohol in "The Greatest Gift of All" (1993). *Magnet Hospitals, Attraction, and Retention of Professional Nurses*

PHASE ONE: PROJECTING THE PLAN

Write

☐ Make a commitment to write a journal article for publication (Chapter 1)

☐ Write about your writer's blocks – a five-minute free flow (Chapter 1)

☐ Generate ideas for articles (Chapter 2)

☐ Select an idea about which to write (Chapter 2)
I will write about _____

☐ Describe your purpose in writing your article (Chapter 3)
I will write the article to _____

☐ Describe an organizing framework that might work for your article (Chapters 3 and 7)
The organizing framework I will use is _____

☐ Write three working titles. Choose the one that best describes your article (Chapter 3)
1. _____
2. _____
3. _____

Market

☐ Describe your desired readers (Chapter 3). Include the setting in which they work, their specialties, and what they probably want or need to know about your topic.

Setting _____

Specialty _____

Desired information _____

Task and Timeline (Chapter 3)

What three journals that are appropriate to your topic does your desired audience read? (Chapter 3)

1. _____

2. _____

3. _____

What general journals do you think might be good target journals for your article? (Chapter 3)

1. _____

2. _____

3. _____

Figure 3.1. The writing plan based on the Writing and Marketing Process (© 1995, Dowdney & Sheridan).

What specialty publications do you think might be a good target journal for your article? (Chapter 3)

1. _____

2. _____

3. _____

Tasks

	Tasks	Begin date	End date
1	Decide to write		
2	Generate ideas		
3	Develop a plan		
4	Select a target publication		
5	Gather information		
6	Organize the content		
7	Communicate with editors		
8	Write the manuscript		
9	Revise the manuscript		
10	Prepare and send the manuscript		

PHASE TWO: COMPLETING THE PLAN

As you read chapters 4 through 10, complete the exercises in those chapters and check them below.

- ☐ Complete several Target Journal Analysis Forms (Chapter 4)
- ☐ Complete the selection section of the Target Journal Selection and Tracking Form (Chapter 4)
- ☐ Gather information about your topic. Complete your literature search and/or plan and schedule your interview (Chapter 5)
- ☐ Complete the ten steps to organize your manuscript (Chapter 6)
- ☐ Design a Sun Diagram for your query letter (Chapter 7)
- ☐ Write a lead for your article (Chapter 7)
- ☐ Write and send a query letter (Chapter 7)

PHASE THREE: ACTING ON EDITORIAL RESPONSES

Upon response to your query letter (Chapter 7)
- ☐ If rejected, gather recommendations for improvement, revise your query letter, and find new target journals
- ☐ If you do not receive a response, call the editor or send a follow-up letter with the original query letter attached
- ☐ If accepted, write the article (Chapter 8)

- ☐ Edit the article (Chapter 9)
- ☐ Seek recommendations from your colleagues (Chapter 10)
- ☐ Prepare to send the manuscript (Chapter 10)
- ☐ Send the manuscript (Chapter 10)

PHASE FOUR: BEGINNING A NEW PLAN

- ☐ Take out your idea file and select a topic for your next article.

Figure 3.1. *(continued)*

(McClure, Poulin, Sovie & Wandelt, 1983) presents examples of success-ful hospitals. Margaret Sovie (1984) picked up on this theme in "The Eco-nomics of Magnetism."

Another purpose you may have for writing an article is to document or provide a history of an institution, organization, process, product, or pro-cedure, or to review history to learn from it. Hospice, a current popular subject, has its origins in the days of the Crusades. In "Hospice: Looking Back," the author presented this history, thus adding depth to our hospice perception (Hagemaster, 1985). Martha Coursin took an interesting light approach to a historical article in "Reflections: The Good New Days in OB," moving quickly from past to present to future (Coursin, 1984).

To give an opinion or share a viewpoint on an issue in nursing may be another purpose for writing. "Hospital Supported Child Care" (Chabin, 1983); "Getting Doctors to Listen" (Kennedy, 1984); and "How Much is a Nurses' Job Really Worth?" (Brett, 1983) are examples.

To cause readers to think or take action after analyzing facts, trends or events is an additional reason for writing. Examples of this are: "Strate-gies for Ending Wage Discrimination in Nursing" (Moskowitz, 1984); "Reducing Restraints: Impact on Staff Attitudes" (Werner, Cohen, Mans-field, Koroknay, & Braun, 1994); and "Crisis in Long Term Care" (Har-rington, 1985).

As nursing care becomes increasingly complex, articles adapting a gen-eral procedure to a specific topic are welcomed by specialty journal edi-tors. "Sleepless Nights: Obstructive Sleep Apnea in the Pediatric Patient" (Spahis, 1994) and "Behavioral Treatment of Obesity: The Occupational Health Nurses' Role" (Morgan, 1984) are examples of this kind of article.

In addition, sharing an approach to a new problem or dealing with nursing care of a newly diagnosed disease or a disease currently affect-ing more people might be your purpose for writing. In the past, Legion-naire's Disease, bulimia, and anorexia nervosa have all fallen into this category. Later, readers have wanted to know more about genital herpes and toxic shock syndrome as the incidence of these diseases rose. In May 1983, *Heart and Lung* carried "Genital Herpes: An Epidemic Disease" (Couch, Jarratt, Greenberg, & Jackson). In this decade, articles such as "Bugs and Drugs: Antibiotic resistance in the 1990's" (Rickman, 1994) are welcomed by editors.

Your purpose may be to show applications of nursing processes, theo-ries, models, frameworks, or techniques. Examples include "Putting Orlando's Theory into Practice" (Schmieding, 1984) and "Using Orem's Theory: A Plan for All Seasons" (Herrington & Houston, 1984).

You may wish to share patient teaching tools such as "A Teaching book-let for Patients receiving Mantle Field Irradiation" (Gomez, 1995) or "A Discharge Tool for Teaching Parents to Monitor Infant Apnea at Home" (Graber & Balas-Stevens, 1984).

Perhaps you would like to clarify nursing implications related to other disciplines such as surgery or medicine. An example is "Putting the Bite on Mandibular Deficiency" (Angelini & Schmidt, 1984), which explains the procedure and also emphasizes nursing responsibilities in preoperative teaching and postoperative observation for airway obstruction.

As nurse educators integrate education and nursing practice, they have unique approaches they can use in manuscripts. Two authors who do this well are Michael A. Tarcinale and Jay Breyer in "Adult Learning Principles—Basis for Educating the Burn Nurse" (Tarcinale, 1983) and "Setting Passing Scores: A Procedure for Determining Passing Scores on an Examination Using a Criterion-Referenced Methodology" (Breyer, 1983).

Similarly, nurse administrators produce useful articles that integrate management theories with nursing practice in order to convince nurse administrators to use effective management principles. In the book *The New Nurse Manager: A Guide to Management Development* (1984), authors Sheridan, Bronstein, and Walker adapt numerous management theories, models, and principles to nursing practice. The book covers a wide range of topics such as leadership style, negotiating, conflict management, coaching, and organizational development.

Using another body of knowledge in the nursing setting is essential to keep the profession in touch with the thoughts and trends in the rest of the world. Marlene Kramer is exemplary in this, as her book *Reality Shock* (1974), now a classic, followed quickly on the heels of *Future Shock* (Toffler, 1971), presenting current research on this related and timely topic. Another example of relating nonnursing bodies of knowledge to nursing is "Fit to Fly," which addresses the physiological stress of air travel and is written by experienced flight nurses (Saletta, Behler, & Charmings, 1984). More current is the adaptation of the chaos theme, popular in the business literature, in "Thriving on Chaos' Work in Health Services Management" (Mollohan, 1994).

To provide an overview or roundup of information on a topic such as salaries "1993 Earnings Survey: How Your Fringe Benefits Stock Up" (Lippman, 1993), or "Where Hospitals Fall Short" (Lee, 1984) is another purpose you may have for writing. Overview articles often require some type of literature survey to gather information.

Sharing a new approach to an old problem is a further reason for writing. Even articles about the "same old problems" in nursing are welcome when you can give new solutions. Examples include: "Job Satisfaction: Assumptions and Complexities" (Larson et al., 1984); "Evaluating Disposable Briefs . . . Treating Incontinence" (Boulton & Kazemi, 1984); and "Effectiveness of a Handwashing Program" (Day, 1993).

Be clear about your purpose in writing an article. Define your article's purpose by saying, "I want to (convince), (inform), (explain), or (describe) . . .". For example, authors may have said: "I want to convince nurses of the problems nursing diagnosis creates by setting up a power relationship in which the nurse is the expert and the patient merely a diagnostic category" when planning their article on "The Problem of Professional Labeling" (Hagey & McDonough, 1984, pp. 151–157). "Where Will You Work Tomorrow" (Hurley, 1994) confronts the '90s downsizing and layoff issues with sound advice for nurses. "We want to inform nurses about the trends that may affect nursing's future" must have been the intention of Kathleen Andreoli and Leigh Anne Musser when planning their article "Trends That May Affect Nursings' Future" (1985). "We want to learn from the Cyprus health policies and strategies that emphasize the value of the individual in a caring family" must have been a motivator in the writing and publication of "The Role of the O. R. Nurse in Cyprus" (Cristadoulou & Kyriakidou, 1994).

If you have difficulty writing your manuscript's purpose, you need to define it more clearly. What do you want to happen to your reader? What would be a desirable outcome of your article? Do you want nurses to make a change in nursing practice? Would your article provide a good solution to a common problem? Would it cause a reader to write a congressman or other government official? Would your article cause the reader to better understand a nursing issue? Would your article help a reader apply a useful educational or administrative theory to nursing practice? Determining desired outcomes will help you define your purpose in writing. In defining your purpose, consider why someone would read an article on the topic you have selected.

The Organizing Framework

All manuscripts need to be organized around a theme with subtopics arranged sequentially and, within these, individual paragraph units developed as complete thoughts. This begins with an organizing idea:

> An organizing idea is a one-sentence summary of the main idea to be dealt with in the paper. Such an organizing idea not only summarizes what the paper is about, but it also shows the restriction on the topic . . . the main function of the organizing idea is to designate your subject and to provide you with a rudder for maintaining its restriction and focus. (Gelderman, 1984, p. 17)

The organizing idea becomes the core of an organizing framework for your manuscript. Strunk and White (1979) call the framework a design. They suggest that writers choose a suitable design and stay with that design throughout the manuscript:

> A basic structural design underlies every kind of writing. The writer will in part follow this design, in part deviate from it, according to his skill, his needs, and the unexpected events that accompany the act of composition. Writing, to be effective, must follow closely the thoughts of the writer, but not necessarily in the order in which those thoughts occur . . . in most cases planning must be a deliberate prelude to writing. The first principle of composition, therefore, is to foresee or determine the shape of what is to come and pursue that shape. (Strunk & White, 1979, p. 15).

Frameworks are your manuscript's backbone or its organizational design. They give order to manuscripts and hold them together. Often they provide the article's subheadings. Although Chapter Six covers this topic in more depth, at this point frameworks are introduced so that you can make a decision about how you might organize your material.

All articles have the basic organizing framework of beginning, middle, and end. The beginning entices readers to begin the article and is called "the lead" or "the hook." Effective leads are essential because not all readers are as interested in your ideas as you are. Therefore, you must create interest by promising the reader new insights, ideas, facts, entertainment, or news. Some types of leads include startling facts or shocking statements, quotations, questions, comparisons, generalizations, narrative, description, summary of the article, or information including who, what, when, where, why, and how.

The middle of the article must have another organizational plan that logically orders this larger body of information. This is the organizing framework explained above. In addition to beginning, middle, and end, you need to use other organizing frameworks to organize the body (middle) of the manuscript. They can be as general as the nursing process or as detailed as the nursing research process. In the latter framework, a copy of the journal in which you would like to publish the article will clearly show the outline your manuscript must follow if each article in that publication follows the same format.

However, most journals have several article types. Even *Nursing Research* varies the format from article to article, often combining one or two of the research steps where necessary for conciseness. This journal also carries articles on nursing theory, a methodology section, guest editorial, and a comments section, all of which necessarily follow non-research formats.

Organizing frameworks can be as simple as a question title with an answer article. Rephrasing your idea as a question will also help you focus your idea. Barbara Brown (1983) organized "What Is Business Savvy?" by asking the question and organizing the body based on the answer. The elements of business savvy could be used as subheadings.

You also may use a series of questions and answers as your organizing framework, as in "15 Problems in Patient Education and Their Solutions" (Rankirt & Duffy, 1984). Margaret Sovie (1985) also used a clear organizing framework by identifying and using the 10 components of a strategic action plan for managing nursing resources as the major subheadings for "Managing Nursing Resources in a Constrained Economic Environment."

Some frameworks evolve naturally when you use the diagramming technique in Chapter Six on organizing. Another way to organize your material may be to use all or part of the nursing process (Yura & Walsh, 1978), as do the authors of "The Role of Nursing in Bereavement: Assessment, Planning, and Intervention Strategies to Improve Care for the Grieved" (Martinson, Dimond, MacElveen-Hoehn, & Barrell, 1984).

Case studies and historical or development approaches are also useful organizing frameworks. Nursing articles may use theoretical frameworks or conceptual models. One participant in our writing class used Sister Callista Roy's (1976) model of adaptation to relate a unique case study about an OB patient.

Fill in an organizing framework on your Plan. If you are not sure which framework to choose, try any one that might work and revise your choice later, if necessary, as you read Chapter Six. Selecting and using frameworks are difficult parts of the Writing Process. However, without this step your chances of writing a publishable article are slim.

The Working Title

After you define your purpose, organizing idea, and organizing framework, select a working title. If your topic is "illnesses people get from too much heat" and your purpose is to describe to nurses how to prevent heat-related illnesses, then your organizing framework might be normal to abnormal: "What is a normal response to the heat?," then "What is the response of the high-risk person?," followed by a description of heat-related illnesses and how to prevent them. In actuality, your working title might be "Preventing Heat-Related Illness." The authors used the following subheadings: The High-Risk Person; Normal Response to Heat; Types of Heat-Related Illnesses; and Prevention and Interventions in their article "Heat and Heat-Related Illness" (Boyd, Shurett, Coburn, 1981).

If your target journal is *Infection Control*, you may want a title such as "Surgical Scrub and Skin Disinfection" (Ayliffe, 1984); or even "Current

Handwashing Issues" (Larson, 1984). If you are describing a study on handwashing that you may want to publish in *American Journal of Infection Control* or *Nursing Research,* perhaps your title would be "Duration of Handwashing in Intensive Care Units: A Descriptive Study" (Quraishi, McGuckin, & Blais, 1984).

For a contemporary journal such as *RN,* a positive, catchy title may be appropriate, such as "Fired! What to Do if It Happens to You" (Campbell, 1984) and "Nursing Still Considered 'Women's Work'," an article based on a survey by the Sonoma County Commission on the Status of Women (1984).

However, more scientific journals such as *Oncology Nursing Forum* often publish articles with more complete and precise titles, usually research-based, such as "The Effects of Infusion Methods on Platelet Count, Morphology, and Corrected Count Increment in Children with Cancer: In Vitro and In Vivo Studies" (Norville et al., 1994). *The Journal of Heart and Lung: Critical Care* usually expects a more complete, formal title, such as "Ambulation after Sheath Removal: A Comparison of 6 and 8 Hours of Bedrest after Sheath Removal in Patients Following a PTCA Procedure" (Fowlow, Price & Furg, 1995).

Remember, the title is often the only information that gives clues to your reader about your topic. Even for general nursing journals, you should write a title that conveys the article's content. Titles also guide library searchers who are scanning the literature; thus, titles are the most widely consulted part of an article. Because indices and other writers' reference lists use manuscript titles, the title you select must capture the manuscript's essence, attract the reader's attention, and indicate what the article is about. Good examples are "Self Directed Teams: Your Role" (Sheridan, 1994) in *Staff Development Insider* and "Assisting with Career Changes in Nursing" (Cummings, 1994) in the same publication; "The Patient Self-Determination Act: Sources of Concern for Nurses" (Mezey, Evans, Golub, Murphy, & White, 1994) and "Will You Recognize these Oncological Crises?" (Schweid, Etheredge, Werner-McCullough, 1994).

The purpose of the working title at this point is to keep you focused as you develop the article. It states the theme. Consider several possible working titles and select the one that best describes the article you plan to write.

The Target Audience

Whether or not your manuscript is publishable in a journal depends on how well you can fulfill the needs of the publication's target audience; the group of readers toward whom you direct your manuscript is its target audience. Characteristics of the target audience are similarities in specialty, health care setting, educational level, level of knowledge about the content of the article, values, interests, profession, needs, or some combination of these factors.

Readers want to learn about new developments, concepts, and approaches to existing practices. They also want to become better informed through new interpretations and opinions. For this information, they read articles such as "HIV Vaccine Trials: A Report From the Front" (Zurlinden & Verheggen, 1994); "More about Nurse Practitioners" (Creighton, 1984).

Readers want to learn how to become more effective professionals. This subject is continually addressed in the nursing literature from a variety of perspectives such as "The Road to Professional Growth" (Levenstein, 1984), written to nurse managers; and "Professionalism among Nurse Educators" (Schriner & Harris, 1984), written to nurses in education.

You might try writing book reviews for a journal or personnel organization, or write news briefs for your hospital or nursing association newsletter. This is a good way to break into writing, and you can learn to be aware of audience interest by being physically close to your readers.

Readers want to obtain specialized information. In "What Makes a Good Story?" (Allen, 1981), the author shared the editor's perspective:

> So how do we choose what is a story and what is not? The main criteria is how many of our readers it will interest. If the story is relevant to only one nurse, then it might be mentioned, but not in any detail. If I think it has wider interest, we will probably follow it up. Ideally every story would make all our readers sit up and think 'that affects me.' (p. 67)

You can determine your manuscript's target audience by visualizing your reader:

> Where is she? She doesn't always read at 10 in the morning, fresh and alert, comfortably seated at a desk, with no distractions. Your reader may be commuting on a train or bus or plane. She may be at lunch, with a sandwich, in a coffee shop or nurses' lounge. And the reader that I always visualize is the one, often like myself, coming home in the middle hours of the evening after a day of decision making and dealing with routines and conflicts, drained and weary. You must entice these readers—catch their attention and hold their interest—if you want to get your message across. (Luckraft, 1982, p. 6)

Answer the question: Who would benefit from reading my manuscript? In nursing journals, the answer may be defined by various roles: clinical, educational, or administrative. These groups are divided into clinical specialists such as cardiovascular or oncological nurses. Clinical nurses can also be divided by the setting in which they work, such as corporate or nonprofit hospital settings, industrial settings, or extended care facilities.

Nurse educators can be divided by setting—hospital, college, or diploma programs, and also by undergraduate or graduate levels. Articles appealing to one group of educators may hold little interest for another group. For example, nurses teaching continuing education might want to read "Moving into Nursing Management: A CE Video Program for RNs" in the *Journal of Continuing Education in Nursing* (Zeimann, 1984), whereas baccalaureate instructors in academia would probably prefer "Senior Students' Experience in Primary Nursing" (Horacek, 1984).

Nurse managers may want to read according to levels—first line managers are interested in a different kind of article than are nurses in nursing administration. For example, a new first line manager might want to read "How Does Your Unit Operate?" (Valentine, 1983). Nurse administrators might be more attracted to articles focusing on planning and decision making. These differences in management levels are decreasing and melding into new titles, such as service line leaders, which blend not only levels but disciplines.

Various combinations of the above are also possible. For example, some articles appeal to nurse educators who teach nursing administration; some appeal to first line nurse managers who manage specialty clinicians, such as emergency nurses or home health nurses. Again, roles are meeting in the continuum of care. However, the audience of the journal is key. For example, if a home health nurse wanted to write for the emergency nurses' publication, the article might be "Follow-up on Your Home Health Patient Post E.D. Visit."

In analyzing your target audience, consider the variety of generalist journals such as *American Journal of Nursing, Nursing,* or *RN.* The following four articles could have been published in *AJN*s or specialty journals. Where do you think each was published? (See the end of this chapter for the answers.)

1. "Violence in the ED: How To Stop It Before It Starts"
2. "The 10 Prescription Drugs Most Toxic to Children"
3. "Effects of Low-Dose Heparin on Failure of Intravenous Infusions in Children"
4. "Coping with Urinary Incontinence: Development and Testing of a Scale"

What you are defines what you are best prepared to write about. Remember, write what you know best. If you work in gerontology and your topic deals with nursing care for elderly patients, the topic would interest nurses in general as well as public health and gerontological nurses. In addition, depending on the specific topic, perhaps it would also interest operating room, emergency room, or student nurses, or specialists such as oncology nurses or cardiac nurses. However, you would write your article quite differently for each of these groups.

The Target Journals

The journal in which you would like to have your finished article published depends on your target audience. You can probably select several journals that your target audience reads. If you are writing for nurses in your own specialty, list journals that you read. (Appendix 3 has an extensive list of journals from which you can select a target.) You can find lists of journals in the front of nursing indices.

For this phase of the Writing Process, define your target market on a gut level. What journals are read by the nurses you want to read your article? Later chapters address this topic in more depth, especially Chapter Four. You can review your choice in light of specific criteria, and you can refine your marketing choices as your article develops.

The Time Schedule

Even at this early phase of the Process, planning includes making a commitment to yourself and, if applicable, your co-author(s). If you do not break up the tasks and set target dates, you will have a good chance of falling into one of the most common blocks to writing—procrastination. If procrastination has been a problem for you in the past, ask editors for deadlines:

> A deadline will spur you to complete the project. It will also provide a feeling of value for what you are creating, and will enhance your feeling of accomplishment once you finish a manuscript. If the editor doesn't set a deadline for you, set one for yourself. (Banks, 1984, p. 33)

Set up a rough timeline using the steps of the Writing Process chapters as your tasks. Plan to do one step (one chapter) each day or each week. Fill in the dates in pencil next to the table of contents; then transfer them to your calendar.

> Set goals within goals. Don't take on the entire project at once. Break it up into manageable sections by assigning yourself goals of a certain number of words or pages to be completed. After each goal is reached, assign yourself a new goal. This step-by-step method makes a deadline less imposing, and a large project seem smaller. (Banks, 1984, p. 33)

If your target journal is *Nursing Research,* you may need to add several tasks to your list in your Writing Plan, such as planing and conducting the research study and analyzing findings. If your framework is question-and-answer based on interviews with experts, you will need to add the tasks of scheduling, developing, and conducting your interviews.

If you are collaborating with another author to write an article, you may want to use Figure 3.2, "The General Planning Form for Collaborative Article Writing." Set up a series of meeting dates or telephone conferences, and fill in dates and tasks for your meetings. Adjust the Planning Form after you use it a few times so that it is realistic. Do not set the dates so close together that you always miss them—missing planned sessions will kill your writing motivation.

If you collaborate to write a book, look at Figure 3.3, Specific Planning Form for Collaborative Book Writing. We have filled in parts of this form to illustrate some of the details involved in revising this book.

Finding Time to Write

How do busy nurse leaders fit writing into their schedules? Where do they write? Selected nurse authors gave the following responses to our survey question (Sheridan & Dowdney, 1984):

GENROSE J. ALFANO: I write mostly at home—usually about one or two hours for length of actual writing periods. I spend a great deal of time writing 'in my head' for more. It's sporadic rather than systematic, and I usually need deadlines.

IRENE M. BOBAK: I write at home in every space; this decreases sleep and social life.

BARBARA J. BROWN: I write at home—never find time at work. At least one time per week, 5–6 hours at the desk. Also early morning several times per week before 6:00 A.M.

LUTHER CHRISTMAN: On weekends; I usually write in the early morning.

RHEBA DE TORNYAY: I write at home. It depends on other activities in my life as an administrator, but on the average, I write one day each weekend.

DOROTHY J. DEL BUENO: I work at writing in the morning in my own office, not my faculty office.

DONNA DIERS: I don't schedule it; I do it all the time: nights, weekends, mornings off, on airplanes, and in hotel rooms. I do all my writing at home—it's too busy in the office. I need a period of time to write—3 to 4 hours minimum unless I'm editing, and then it goes faster.

Topic of article
First author
Second author
Third author
Fourth author
Date to complete manuscript

Tasks (Description/Comments)	Person Responsible	Dates	Completed
1			
2			
3			
4			
5			
6			
7			
8			
9			
10			

Figure 3.2. General Planning Form for collaborative article writing (© 1995, Dowdney & Sheridan).

VERNICE FERGUSON: I write at home with maximum periods of three hours at any given time. My best writing precedes deadlines, generally 1–3 days before a deadline.

BARBARA STEVENS BARNUM: I never schedule my writing. I write when I have something to say. (I also write if I have taken on a commitment, e.g., when I must prepare a speech in written copy.)

MARGRETTA M. STYLES: I attempt to devote at least one hour a day to writing during the normal work week. This occurs between 4–6 A.M. On weekends I spend longer periods, and on sabbaticals 8–10 hours/day. I write at home, comfortably seated on a sofa in the study, using a lap board.

DUANE D. WALKER: I schedule myself on my work calendar. When possible, I take a day off to write.

Section	Description/ Comments		Responsible Author & Date Completed		Dates Sent to Other Author	
			Sheridan	Dowdney	To other author	To original author
Title page 1	Add award		Publisher	Publisher	Publisher	Publisher
Biographies		3/95	7/94	7/94		
Title page 2			Publisher	Publisher	Publisher	Publisher
Copyright			Publisher	Publisher	Publisher	Publisher
Dedication		3/95	12/94	12/94	12/94	12/94
Continuing ed		3/95	x			
Contents			Publisher	Publisher	Publisher	Publisher
Foreword 1		3/95	x			
Foreword 2		3/95	x			
Preface		3/95	4/95	x		
1: Decide to Write		3/95	x4/95			
2: Generate Ideas		3/95	x4/95			
3: Develop Plan		3/95	x4/95			
4: Select Journal	Ref 86	3/95	4/95	x		
5: Gather Info	Table 5-1	3/95	4/95	x		
6: Organize		3/95	x4/95			
7: Communicate		3/95	x4/95			
8: Write	New technology	3/95	4/95	x		
9: Revise		3/95	4/95	x		
10: Prepare & Send		3/95	4/95	x		
Epilogue			x4/95			
Ap 1: Publications			4/95		7/94	7/94
Ap 2: Associations			4/95		7/94	7/94
Ap 3: Publication			4/95			
Index			Publisher	Publisher	Publisher	Publisher
Survey			x			
Figures (some)			4/95	3-1 3-2 4-1 4-2 5-1 5-2 5-3 10-		

Figure 3.3. Specific Planning Form for collaborative book writing (© 1995, Dowdney & Sheridan).

HELEN YURA: I write at home. I spend a long time thinking, making notes, and outlining. Then I start to write and keep at it until I'm finished. I then let the draft cool a few days; I re-read and make any editorial adjustments needed.

MARY LLOYD ZUSY: I work at home, and usually start around nine in the morning, break for lunch, and work again from about 2:30 P.M. until 4:00 P.M.

Other respondents to our survey make time to write by getting up earlier, going to bed later, or working during their lunch hour. They write on the train or plane, or work on several projects at once in the library. Some dictate their articles into a tape recorder as they drive.

GATHERING INFORMATION

After you draft your Writing Plan, the next step is to gather information. Unless you have been gathering information on your topic in your home library or information files, you will need to visit a library. The purpose is twofold: to search for the appropriate market for your article and to search for content already published on your topic. Information gathering also may include interviewing selected experts.

The next three chapters address gathering information. Beginning at the library, search for your target market. Then, while you are at the library, review content related to your topic. Next, you may want to gather additional information from experts on your topic.

ANSWERS TO QUESTIONS (P. 61)

1. *American Journal of Nursing,* July 1993
2. *American Journal of Nursing,* July 1993
3. *Heart and Lung,* Jan./Feb. 1995
4. *Nursing Diagnosis,* July–Sept. 1994

EXERCISES

1. Describe an organizing framework that might work for your article.
2. Write three working titles that best describe the article you plan to write.

REFERENCES

Allen, M. (1981, May 7). What makes a good story? *Nursing Mirror*, p. 67.

Andreoli, K. G., & Musser, L. A. (1985). Trends that may affect nursing's future. *Nursing and Health Care, 6*(1), 47–51.

Angelini, C., & Schmidt, M. (1984). Putting the bite on mandibular deficiency. *Today's OR Nurse, 6*(6), 14–17.

Ayliffe, G. A. (1984). Surgical scrub and skin disinfection. *Infection Control, 5*(1), 23–27.

Banks, M. A. (1984, July). 10 steps to greater writing productivity. *Writer's Digest*, 33.

Beaudoin, K. (1983). Going the distance with the patient who's a real fighter. *Nursing, 13*(4), 70–75.

Boulton, S. W., & Kazemi, M. J. (1984). Evaluating disposable briefs . . . treating incontinence. *American Journal of Nursing, 84*(11), 1413, 1439.

Boyd, L. T., Shurett, P. H., & Coburn, C. (1981). Heat and heat-related illnesses. *American Journal of Nursing, 81*(7), 1298–1302.

Brett, J. L. (1983). How much is a nurses' job really worth? *American Journal of Nursing, 83*(6), 876–881.

Breyer, F. J. (1983, November). Setting passing scores: A procedure for determining passing scores on an examination using a criterion-referenced methodology. *Nursing and Health Care, 4*(9), 518–522.

Brown, B. S. (1983). What is business savvy? *Nursing Economics, 1*(1), 52–53.

Campbell, L. M. (1984, June). Fired! What to do if it happens to you. *RN, 47*(6), 58–60.

Casey, D. (1993). The greatest gift of all. *American Journal of Nursing, 93*(9), 46–47.

Chabin, M. (1983). Hospital-supported child care. *American Journal of Nursing, 83*(4), 548–552.

Christodoulou, P., & Kyriakidou, S. (1994). The role of the OR nurse in Cyprus. *Today's OR Nurse, 16*(6), 24–26.

Costello, C. (1984). Sally had a drug habit, but I looked the other way. *Nursing Life, 4*(3), 28–29.

Couch, R. B., Jarratt, M. T., Greenberg, S. B., and Jackson, D. (1983). Genital herpes: An epidemic disease. *Heart and Lung, 12*(3), 320–324.

Coursin, M. (1984). The good new days in OB. *American Journal of Nursing, 84*(4), 580.

Creighton, H. (1984). More about nurse practitioners. *Nursing Management, 15*(9), 64–65.

Cummings, C. (1994). Assisting with career changes in nursing. *Nursing Staff Development Insider, 3*(1), 2, 6.

Day, R. A. (1993). Effectiveness of a handwashing program. *Clinical Nursing Research, 2*(1), 24–40.

Fowlow, B., Price, D., & Fung, T. (1995). Ambulation after sheath removal: A comparison of 6 and 8 hours of bedrest after sheath removal in patients following a PTCA procedure. *Heart & Lung: The Journal of Critical Care, 24*(1), 28–37.

Gelderman, C. (1984). *Better writing for professionals.* Glenview, IL: Scott, Foresman & Company.

Gomez, E. G. (1995). A teaching booklet for patients receiving mantle field irradiation. *Oncology Nursing Forum, 22*(1), 121–126.

Graber, H. P., & Balas-Stevens, S. (1984). A discharge tool for teaching parents to monitor infant apnea at home. *American Journal of Maternal/Child Nursing, 9*(3), 178–180.

Guttenberg, R. M. (1983). How to stay cool in a conflict and turn it into cooperation. *Nursing Life, 3*(3), 17–24.

Hagemaster, J. N. (1985). Hospice: Looking back. *Topics in Clinical Nursing, 7*(1), 79–85.

Hagey, R. S., & McDonough, P. (1984). The problem of professional labeling. *Nursing Outlook, 32*(3), 151–157.

Harrington, C. (1985). Crisis in long term care. *Nursing Economics, 3*(1), 15.

Heineken, J., & McCloskey, J. C. (1985, January). Teaching power concepts. *Journal of Nursing Education, 24*(1), 40–42.

Herrington, J. V., & Houston, S. (1984). Using Orem's theory: A plan for all seasons. *Nursing and Health Care, 5*(1), 45–47.

Hinkle, J. L. (1994). Neurotoxins: A neuroscience nursing challenge. *Journal of Neuroscience Nursing, 26*(5), 261–264.

Horacek, L. A. (1984). Senior students' experience in primary nursing. *Journal of Nursing Education, 23*(3), 122–124.

Hurley, M. L. (1994). Where will you work tomorrow? *RN, 57*(8), 36–41.

Huth, E. J. (1982). *How to write and publish papers in the medical sciences.* Philadelphia: ISI Press.

Kennedy, C. W. (1984, May–June). Getting doctors to listen. *Nursing Life, 4*(3), 54–56.

Kramer, M. (1974). *Reality Shock.* St. Louis: C. V. Mosby, 1974.

Larson, E. (1984). Current handwashing issues (Editorial). *Infection Control, 5*(1), 18–22.

Larson, E., Lee, P. C., Brown, M. A., & Shorr, J. (1984). Job Satisfaction: Assumptions and complexities. *Journal of Nursing Administration, 14*(1), 31–38.

Lay, M. M., Wahlstrom, B. J., Duin, A H., Little, S. B., Selfe, C. L., Selzer, J., Rude, C., & Doheny-Farina, S. (1995). *Technical Communication.* Chicago: Richard D. Irwin, Inc.

Lee, A. (1984, April). Where hospitals fall short. *RN, 47*(4), 34–37.

Levenstein, A. (1984). The road to professional growth. *Nursing Management, 15*(7), 60–61.

Lippman, H. (1993). 1993 earnings survey: How your fringe benefits stack up. *RN, 56*(12), 40–45.

Lovett, R. B., Reardon, M. B., Gordon, B. K., & McMillan, S. (1994). Validity and reliability of medical and surgical oncology patient acuity tools. *Oncology Nursing Forum, 21*(10), 1709–1717.

Luckraft, D. (1982, February). Does scholarly writing have to be boring? *Nursing and Healthcare, 3*(2), 67.

Martinson, I. M., Dimond, M., MacElveen-Hoehn, P., & Barrell, L. M. (1984). The role of nursing in bereavement. *The American Journal of Hospice Care, 1*(2), 14–16.

McClure, M. L., Poulin, M. A., Sovie, M. D., & Wandelt, M. A. (1983) *Magnet hospitals, attraction and retention of professional nurses.* Kansas City, MO: American Nurses' Association.

McConnell, P. (1984). Surgery for dental function: The team approach to Le Forte 1 Osteotomy, *Today's OR Nurse, 6*(6), 19–21, 24–25.

McLaughlin, F. E. (1981, May). The publication of nursing research. *The Journal of Nursing Administration, 11,* 38.

Mezey, M., Evans, L., Golub, Z. D., Murphy, E., White, G. B. (1994). The Patient Self-Determination Act: Sources of concern for nurses. *Nursing Outlook, 42*(1), 30–37.

Michaelson, H. B., (1990). *How to write and publish engineering papers and reports.* Phoenix, AZ: Oryx.

Miller, K. P. & Dickerson, J. K. (1984). Should critical care nurses participate in pharmacologic research? *Dimensions of Critical Care Nursing, 3*(3), 162–70.

Miller, D., & Miller, H. W. (1995). A nurse's guide to tube feeding. *RN, 58*(1), 44–48.

Mitchell, K. (1984). Protecting children's rights during research. *Pediatric Nursing, 10*(1), 9–10.

Mollohan, C. J. (1994). "Thriving on chaos" works in health services management. *Nursing Management, 25*(5), 80B, 80D, 80F.

Morgan, J. (1984). Behavioral treatment of obesity: The occupational health nurses' role. *Occupational Health Nursing, 32*(6), 312.

Moskowitz, S. (1984). Strategies for ending wage discrimination in nursing. *Nursing Economics, 2*(1), 25.

Norville, R., Hinds, P., Wilimas, J., Fairclough, D., Fischl, S., & Kunkel, K. (1994). The effects of infusion methods on platelet count, morphology, and corrected count increment in children with cancer: In vitro and in vivo studies. *Oncology Nursing Forum, 21*(10), 1669–1706.

Nursing still considered "women's work." (1984). *RN, 47*(6), 70.

O'Brien, M. E. (1983). Reaching the migrant worker. *American Journal of Nursing, 83*(6), 895.

O'Connor, A. B. (1980, April). "Who, me? write?" *Today's OR Nurse, 2*(2), 22–23.

Pierson, M. A., & Boosinger, J. K. (1984). Follow-up of cardiac pacemaker recipients: A pilot study. *Heart and Lung, 13*(4), 431–435.

Prakasamma, M. (1984). A study of yoga as a nursing intervention in the care of patients with pleural effusion. *Journal of Advanced Nursing, 9*(2), 127–133.

Quarles, A., Williams, R. D., Hoyle, D. A., Brimeyer, M., & Williams, A. R. (1994). Mothers' intention, age, education and the duration and management of breastfeeding. *Maternal-Child Nursing Journal, 22*(3), 102–108.

Quraishi, Z. A., McGuckin, M., & Blais, F. X. (1984). Duration of handwashing in intensive care units: A descriptive study. *American Journal of Infection Control, 12*(2), 83–87.

Rankirt, S., & Duffy, K. (1984, April). 15 problems in patient education and their solutions. *Nursing, 14*(6), 67–72.

Rickman, L. S. (1994). Bugs and drugs: Antibiotic resistance in the 1990s. *Today's OR Nurse, 16*(5), 7–12.

Roy, C. (1976). *Introduction to nursing: An adaptation model.* Englewood Cliffs, NJ: Prentice-Hall.

Saletta, A. L., Behler, D. M., & Charmings, P. A. (1984). Fit to fly. *American Journal of Nursing, 84*(4), 462–465.

Sargis, N. M. (1985). Collective bargaining: Serving the common good in a crisis. *Nursing Management, 16*(2), 23–27.

Schmieding, N. J. (1984). Putting Orlando's theory into practice. *American Journal of Nursing, 84*(6), 759–761.

Schriner, J., & Harris, I. (1984). Professionalism among nurse educators. *Journal of Nursing Education, 23*(6), 252–258.

Schweid, L., Etheredge, C., & Werner-McCullough, M. (1994). Will you recognize these oncological crises? *RN, 57*(9), 22–29.

Sheridan, D. R. (1994). Self-directed teams: Your role. *Nursing Staff Development Insider, 3*(1), 1, 7.

Sheridan, D. R. Bronstein, J. E., & Walker, D. D. (1984). *The new nurse manager: A guide to management development.* Gaithersburg, MD: Aspen.

Sheridan, D. R., & Dowdney, D. L. (1984). *Survey of selected nurse authors.* Unpublished work.

Sovie, M. D. (1984, March–April). The economics of magnetism. *Nursing Economics, 2*(2), 85–92.

Sovie, M. (1985). Managing nursing resources in a constrained economic environment. *Nursing Economics, 3*(2), 85.

Spahis, J. (1994). Sleepless nights: Obstructive sleep, apnea in the pediatric patient. *Pediatric Nursing, 20*(5), 469–472.

Stein, J. (1983). Sheila Barnes had a knack for making me feel awkward. *Nursing Life, 2*(3), 1.

Strunk, W., & White, E. B. (1979). *The elements of style.* New York: Macmillan.

Tarcinale, M. A. (1983). Adult learning principles—Basis for educating the burn nurse. *Journal of Burn Care and Rehabilitation, 4*(1), 19–23.

Toffler, A. (1971). *Future shock.* New York: Bantam.

Valentine, P. E. B. (1983). How does your unit operate? *Nursing Leadership, 6*(2), 40–43.

Watson-Rouslin, V., & Peck, J. M. (1985, March). Double time. *Writer's Digest*, 32–34.

Weiner, E. E., & Weiner, D. L. (1983, May). Understanding the use of basic statistics in nursing research. *American Journal of Nursing, 83*(5), 770–774.

Werner, P., Cohen-Mansfield, J., Koroknay, V., & Braun, J. (1994). Reducing restraints: Impact on staff attitudes. *Journal of Gerontological Nursing, 20*(12), 19–24.

Yura, H. & Walsh, M. B. (1978). *The nursing process.* New York: Appleton, Century, Crofts.

Zeimann, L. K. (1984). Moving into nursing management: A CE video program for RNs. *Journal of Continuing Education in Nursing, 15*(5), 164–167.

Zurlinden, J., & Verheggen, R. (1994). HIV vaccine trials: A report from the front, *RN, 57*(1), 36–40.

4

Select a Target Journal

Before you write your article or query letter to inquire about editorial interest, and even before you make a final decision on your article's subject, analyze the journals you think will be interested in publishing your article. In the previous chapter you generated multiple article ideas; in this chapter you will learn how to analyze the relevant publishing market and select target journals that "fit" your article.

Each journal has a theme and audience, a style, and a preferred type of content and format. In other words, each journal addresses the needs of a particular audience in a particular manner. For example, *Health Education* focuses on health education and educators rather than on clinical aspects of the field. You need to understand a journal's identity even before you write your article. One editor advised that you do your homework. Know the journal you're submitting to and the types of articles it publishes.

Because editors will not consider even an excellent article if it is sent to the wrong journal, never send an article to a journal editor without reviewing at least one recent copy of that journal. Review back issues to see what the journal has recently covered; look for different angles.

One nursing journal editor said she can usually tell immediately when an author has not even seen a copy of her journal. It makes her angry that the author expects her to invest her time reviewing the manuscript when the author did not even invest the time to review the journal. This editor, who is usually willing to help new writers, said that she does not try to work with these authors.

Besides getting a better understanding of the journal, reviewing the publication before submitting your query letter or manuscript can give you a better idea of the audience that the journal serves. This will increase your chances of an acceptance.

ANALYZING PUBLICATIONS

Although many books tell you to read a publication before sending a manuscript, few tell you how to analyze a publication to properly prepare your manuscript. Reading is not enough. You need to analyze the journal to write an article the editor and the readers desire.

Some of the factors to consider in analysis include theme and audience, style and tone, structure and organizational framework, and use of illustrative materials. The Target Journal Market Analysis Form (Figure 4.1) will help you analyze and select the journals in which you would like your manuscript published. Once you analyze a publication, save the completed form in a journal file for future reference. Fill in these forms as you scan journals.

Journal Theme and Audience

Successful writers are aware of the differing audiences and themes of various journals. A journal's theme tells what a journal is about. The audience is the reader. Each journal has a theme and a target audience. For example, *AACN Clinical Issues in Critical Care Nursing* is the publication of the American Association of Critical Care Nurses. It is published for critical care nurses, pediatric practitioners, educators, managers, and other members of the critical care community. It presents subjects of interest to nurses working in or managing critical care environments.

Nursing Research welcomes manuscripts of relevance and interest to those concerned with the conduct or results of nursing research. *Perioperative Nursing Quarterly* provides nurses and allied health care professionals with information that increases their knowledge and skills in various roles in operating room nursing. It also presents educational resources for staff development activities and classroom instruction. *Imprint*, published by the National Student Nurses Association, publishes general nursing articles of interest to student nurses. For example, "Student of Nursing. . . . Student of Life" is an article about a nursing student's first experience with a homosexual client, followed by information about this "Invisible minority" and "concept of family" (Andrews, 1984).

Your selected topic points the direction for beginning your target journal search. To find the appropriate journal, your topic must match a particular journal's theme. For example, Jill Morgan's article, "Nutritional Assessment of Critically Ill Patients" (1984) matches the critical care theme of *Focus on Critical Care*, as does "Death on a Daily Basis" by Janean Woods in the same issue. The titles of these articles match the journal's title, and, therefore, the theme.

Often you can guess the theme from the journal's name. Without looking at a copy of the journal, however, you would not know if the editors also considered general nursing articles. In other words, because the audience is essentially critical care nurses, is the publication theme limited to articles about critical care, or is it also open to general articles that might interest critical care nurses?

Nursing 95 focuses on the clinical, patient-care side of nursing. We stress the teaching of hands-on skills and procedures, and we address legal, ethical, and professional issues of nursing as well. We publish feature articles and departments plus special sections for particular groups of nurses, such as critical care and long-term-care nurses.

Nursing 95 is a how-to journal, full of hands-on, practical articles. We look for the voice of experience from authors. We're also interested in articles that help our readers deal with problems in their professional lives. We're always interested in taking a look at manuscripts that fall into the following categories:

Clinical articles describing particular diseases, disorders, or conditions, with the emphasis on relevant nursing care. Also, clinical articles focusing on specific assessment techniques, such as assessing heart sounds.

Drug articles focusing on important nursing considerations related to preparing and administering drugs, potential adverse reactions, and careful evaluation of patient response.

Charting/documentation articles that help nurses do this vital but burdensome task more accurately and efficiently.

Emotional problems that patients or their families encounter, such as anger or grief, and how nurses can help them cope.

Legal problems nurses face in their daily work, concerning such things as floating, confidentiality, and informed consent.

Ethical dilemmas nurses play a role in resolving, such as terminal weaning or reporting an impaired colleague.

Difficult or challenging cases that require good nursing skills, teamwork, and resourcefulness.

The Guidelines for *Nursing 95* recommend that you "Write for experienced nurses who give direct patient care. Although most of our readers are medical/surgical nurses, we also have many specialty nurses, including those from critical care and emergency departments."

From *Nursing 95,* Writer's guidelines. Reprinted with permission of Springhouse Corporation.

THEME

Publication name and date _____

Journal theme. Check all that apply.
- ☐ General nursing
- ☐ Specialty (cardiovascular etc.)
- ☐ In-house (newsletter)
- ☐ State nursing publication
- ☐ Other _____

Journal type. Check all that apply.
- ☐ General
- ☐ Scholarly
- ☐ Scientific
- ☐ Research
- ☐ If non-nursing, specify _____

AUDIENCE (READERS OF JOURNAL)

Check all that apply.
- ☐ Clinicians
- ☐ Educators
- ☐ Managers/Administrators
- ☐ Researchers
- ☐ Other _____

Work setting of audience
Check all that apply.
- ☐ In-patient hospital/clinic
- ☐ Out-patient hospital/clinic
- ☐ Community health
- ☐ Home care
- ☐ Physician's office
- ☐ Extended care
- ☐ Industry
- ☐ Other

Title of article _____

STYLE AND TONE

Select 100 words in the article and count the following:
- ☐ Fiction techniques such as stories, dialogue, faction
- ☐ Point of view (first, second, third person)
- ☐ Style and tone (forceful, passive, formal, informal, lively)
- ☐ Adjectives
- ☐ Adverbs
- ☐ Words of more than two syllables
- ☐ Quotes
- ☐ Kinds of transitions
- ☐ Statistics
- ☐ Average sentence length
- ☐ Number of sentences in paragraphs

Figure 4.1. Target Journal Market Analysis Form ((Dowdney & Sheridan © 1996).

STRUCTURE AND ORGANIZATIONAL FRAMEWORK

Number of words in article _____

Reference style (footnotes, bibliography, APA style, Chicago style, etc.)

_____

Framework (look at headings) _____

Number of points covered in article _____

SOURCES/AUTHORITY
Check all that apply.
- ☐ Experts
- ☐ Reports
- ☐ Reference list
- ☐ Computerized databases
- ☐ Other _____

ILLUSTRATIVE MATERIALS
Check all that apply.
- ☐ Charts or graphs
- ☐ Models
- ☐ **Photographs**
- ☐ Color
- ☐ Black-and-white
- ☐ Action
- ☐ Close-up
- ☐ Portrait
- ☐ **Subjects of photographs**
- ☐ Wounds, injuries, or operations
- ☐ People (individuals or groups)
- ☐ Buildings
- ☐ Landscapes
- ☐ Cells
- ☐ Microorganisms

Other _____

PERSONAL APPEAL TO YOU AS AUTHOR
Check all that apply.
- ☐ Refereed publication ___Yes ___No
- ☐ Circulation _____
- ☐ Desire to have article published in journal ___Yes ___No
- ☐ Requirements you would need to meet to be published in this journal

_____
_____
_____

- ☐ Other _____
_____
_____
_____

Figure 4.1. *(continued).*

Specialty journals may or may not include general articles. In *Focus on Critical Care* general articles are included. The issue cited above also includes general nursing articles such as Ellen Rudy's article "A View of Healthcare in the USSR" (1984) and Susan Fetzer-Fowler's "The Future of the Baylor Plan," (1984) an article about innovative scheduling. This specialty journal publishes general interest nursing articles along with articles of special interest to the target audience. Understanding these publishing interests increases the publishing opportunities for your general nursing manuscripts.

In order to discover a journal's specific themes and the scope of acceptable topics, it is essential to review the journal. By reviewing these journal sketches, you may find many more possible publishing opportunities than you had expected.

Because you are responsible for how well your audience understands your message, you must satisfy your reader's need for information more than your own need for self-expression. Concentrate on writing for the needs of specific readers, rather than merely writing about certain subjects. Pinpoint the potential audience by considering the reader's background and orientation. Consider their reading and vocabulary knowledge and their use of your article. Help your readers by defining unfamiliar terms, providing necessary illustrative materials, and writing clearly and concisely.

You will probably be writing in your area of expertise and will be familiar with the journals in your field. A journal's writers often come from that journal's readers, but do not rule out other possibilities. Look over the journal list in Appendix 3 and review a variety of nursing journals in the library to enlarge your repertoire of target journals.

Hundreds of manuscripts and query letters are received by broadscope journals such as *American Journal of Nursing, RN,* and *Nursing.* Therefore, you may increase your chances of acceptance for publication by selecting smaller, newer, or lesser-known publications. State nursing journals are another possibility. You can find out about your state's nursing journal through your state branch of the American Nurses Association. State nursing journals are good targets for articles dealing with local, regional, and state issues such as new state laws on health issues and the implications for nurses.

ORGANIZING FRAMEWORKS

Some journals have one specific framework, outline, or format that must be followed for articles to be accepted for publication. The headings and subheadings are essentially the same, regardless of the article content. This is especially true of research journals. Tornquist (1983) wrote that articles reporting research nearly always contain four parts: Why I Did It (variously named Introduction, Rationale, Background, Problem, or Literature Review); What I Did (Methods); What Happened (Findings or Results); and What It means (Discussion, Implications, Conclusions).

Within some journals a variety of approaches is used such as how to, case study, or nursing process. Many types of organizational frameworks are obvious, such as a question-answer format. In this framework, the question is the article title which the body of the article answers. For example, in *Nursing Quality Connection,* Ellie Green titles her article "When Must Indicators Be Used?" (Green, 1994). Gail Holland Wade also uses this method in her article: "Is Research in the Practice Setting Feasible" (1995).

You can detect other frameworks by looking at headings and subheadings, although sometimes you have to pull an article apart to find the framework. To find the framework, ask yourself: "How is the article organized?" Look at the headings and subheadings. Then ask yourself, "What is the framework that holds the article together?" If you make a habit of examining the organizational framework used each time you look at journal articles, you will begin to get a sense of how to organize your articles. You will begin to know which frameworks particular journals prefer.

Organizing an article is probably the most difficult skill to learn in writing, but it is essential to successful writing. Chapter Six covers this topic in depth. However, while you are searching for a journal's preferred organization within an article, watch for useful frameworks to use in organizing your own articles.

Knowing the types of articles and required formats (such as research) may be sufficient organizational analysis to match the type of article you write for a particular journal. However, a more in-depth analysis and search for frameworks will help you understand the journal's style. The more you understand about a journal's identity, the more likely you are to write an article acceptable for publication in that journal.

Style and Tone

A writer's style is determined by the way the writer transfers thoughts to paper and involves word use, sentences, images, figures of speech, methods of organization, and description. Cardinal Newman said, "Style is a thinking out into language." Aristotle told us where to begin: "A good style must first of all be clear." Goethe said, "If any man wishes to write a clear style, let him first be clear in his thoughts." Shakespeare and Orwell let us know what to avoid: "Plain and not honest is too harsh a style," and "The great enemy of clear language is insincerity."

We built guidelines to help you produce a brisk, interesting style into our Writing Process and presented it throughout this book. Strunk and White captured the essence of style in *The Elements of Style,* which appears in almost every reference list on writing. We believe *The Elements of Style* and a dictionary are required books for all nurse authors.

In "What Do You Mean You Don't Like My Style?" which appeared in *Harvard Business Review,* John S. Fielden analyzed styles used in business communications. Some of his conclusions that follow apply to writing for publication: Each style has an impact on the reader; style communicates to readers almost as much as the content of a message; and style must be altered to suit the circumstances (Fielden, 1982). You express your style through your choice of words, sentences, images, figures of speech, description, and the way you develop your ideas. According to its writer's guidelines, *Nursing 95* has an informal, easy-to-read style. It gives the following specific suggestions about how to achieve that tone:

> Write as if you're talking to the reader. Refer to yourself as "I" and to the reader as "you." So instead of saying "The nurse does this," say "You'd do this next." Use active verbs indicating who is doing what. Instead of saying "the wound is cleaned," say "you clean the wound." Also avoid heavy academic or unnecessarily dense clinical language.
>
> Be specific and give examples for each important point you make. Instead of saying, "Look for signs of infection," for example, include precisely what signs to look for.
>
> Don't try to cover too much. Books might cover topics in great depth, but journals have limited space, so focusing in-depth on one aspect of a patient's problem is best. For example, instead of writing about all types of shock, focus on a specific type, such as septic shock.
>
> Write from your experience. Our readers need to know you've "been there," so give practical advice based on your own experience rather than compiling a research-based article. Use case histories based on real patients you've cared for. (We'll change the names and some details to protect patient anonymity.) (*Nursing 95,* writer's guidelines)

The tone you use in writing expresses your attitude toward your subject and readers. Your tone may be friendly and engaging or hostile and alienating. It can be enthusiastic or skeptical. You set the tone of your manuscript by the attitude you take toward the subject and the techniques you use to make the effect of the writing serious, intimate, or personal.

Viewpoint

Viewpoint is the mind of the character through which you tell a reader a story. Fiction and nonfiction stories use first-person, second-person, and third-person viewpoints. First-person uses the pronoun *I;* the reader experiences events through the main character's or the writer's viewpoint. First-person is especially appropriate for writing opinions, sharing your own perspectives, or writing editorials.

Florence Downs, Editor of *Nursing Research,* wrote in the first person in "News form the Fourth Estate." She shared her perspectives about how the journal had changed over her years as editor. She uses *I* frequently and shows her feelings in her writing. For example, "*I* feel as though it was only yesterday when *I* completed my first issue of *Nursing Research* and said, 'Okay, *I've* proved *I* can do it. *I* quit.'"; and "*I* am, of course, a research buff. There is a certain kind of enchantment in watching the world of nursing research take shape before *my* eyes" (Downs, 1985, p. 3).

The second-person viewpoint uses the pronoun *you;* the author writes directly to the reader. Second-person is a friendly, personal style; we wrote this book using the second-person perspective. Second-person is especially appropriate for teaching, giving advice, and writing "how-to" articles.

In "Tackling Writer's Block," the authors frequently use *you:*

> Make *your* schedule specific . . . schedule *yourself* tightly and fairly, but not slavishly. The point is to help *you* make the best use of *your* talents and the best use of *your* time, not to turn *you* into a robot. . . . Schedule work periods that fit *your* daily schedule, *your* personal work style, and the task at hand (Rosenberg & Lah, 1985, p. 40)

The third-person viewpoint uses the pronouns *he, she,* and *they* or *the writer, the author, the nurse, the researcher*—not *I* or *you.* Third-person is a distant and formal style of writing and is often boring to readers. Research and scientific journal articles are usually written in this style because of the need to appear objective.

Third-person is used in the article "Analysis of Posthospitalization Telephone Survey Data" (Minnick, Roberts, Young, Kleinpell, & Micek, 1995) in which the authors report on a study of 4600 adult patients regarding patient-centered care outcomes. The summary especially characterizes this style: "The authors recommend . . .".

In addition to the above three viewpoints, stories can be written using the objective, subjective, omniscient, multiple character, or detached viewpoint. These viewpoints all overlap first-second-, and third-person viewpoints.

Writers use the objective viewpoint to relate facts and to avoid emotion and opinion. "A Sample of Practical Technology for the Case Manager" (Weed, 1995) and "Clinical Snapshot: Intermittent Claudication" (Dumas, 1995), addressing symptoms and care, are examples of straightforward fact-telling using the objective viewpoint.

Subjective viewpoint allows the writer's thoughts and emotions to be shared. Editorials are often written with a subjective viewpoint. An example of this is "Get One You Can Control," an editorial by Lucie Kelly in *Nursing Outlook* (1985). Kelly, an outstanding nurse writer, often writes thought-provoking editorials in the first person. In this article she addressed dismissal of nurse administrators by beginning with advice she heard one hospital administrator give a colleague who was hiring a director of nursing: "Get one you can control." Her editorial is subjective and controversial . . . and exciting to read. Another example "Peer Review: When Enough is Enough" (Kim, 1994) allows the controversy to show clearly in the title.

Another viewpoint is called "omniscient". It allows authors to relate the perceptions of anyone in the story. The author knows the feelings and thoughts of all characters. Although not commonly used in nonfiction, there might be a time when the author would know the thoughts and feelings of all characters. An example of this is "PKU: A Mother's Perspective." The writer is a mother and a nurse, and because of her dual role she knows and shares both perspectives (Messer, 1985).

Usually, however, you don't know all, as you might in the above dual role or in fiction (where you can make it up). Therefore, you need to ask what the various perspectives on the issue are. This viewpoint is called multiple-character viewpoint. You can use multiple-character viewpoint to tell a story from the perspectives of different relevant people—one at a time. For example, in "Theoretical Foundations of a Prepared Sibling Class," the authors addressed both the child's needs and the parents' needs (Johnsen & Gaspard, 1985).

The detached viewpoint lets readers sense that they are watching the story as it unfolds; the author gives descriptions and impressions, but never through the perception of a character. Or, similar to third-person, the writer addresses himself or herself as "the author" and relates the facts. This informational style never uses *I* or *we*.

Timeliness and Originality

Besides matching the theme, audience, and style and tone, your topic must be timely, original, and not recently covered by the target journal. Journal editors do not want recently covered or out-of-date material. Be sure to review the indices of the past 6 months to one year of a journal's issues to see if the journal published articles on your topic recently.

Another way to determine if journals have recently published on a topic is to look it up in the nursing indices—*Cumulative Index to Nursing and*

Allied Health Literature (the red one) or *International Nursing index* (the green one), both of which are available online. Look for which publications have recently carried an article on your topic. While you check if your topic was covered recently, you can also be gathering content information. Note articles recently written on the topic as a beginning of your literature search. You may want to photocopy the page(s) of the index; the next chapter addresses techniques for library searching.

Timeliness in writing relates to the immediate newsworthiness of a manuscript's topic. For example, a seasonal article dealing with helping patients cope with the "holiday blues" is appropriate for a November–December issue rather than a summer one. Submit seasonal articles at least 6 months in advance of when the material would be appropriate for publication.

Timeliness in nursing journals may be related to how current the issue is that you are addressing. For example, "The Healthcare Industry in the Marketplace: Implications for Nursing" (Sheridan, 1983) used Milton Friedman's economic framework to explore the economic situation as it applied to nursing. Friedman's support of a strong marketplace was reflected in the core of Reaganomics; thus the article needed to be published during this economic trend. Now timely topics sure to be read include: "Surviving a Merger" (Katz & Clemons, 1995); "Trailbreaking—Planning for New Nursing Roles in Managed Care: Information, Innovation and Curriculum Development" (O'Connor, 1993); and "Sexual Harassment: A Concern for Nursing Administrators" (Neubs, 1994).

Originality requires you to stretch and be creative. Originality in writing addresses something new, such as the use of a new product or the effect of a societal, environmental, or political change. More likely, originality is a new approach to something old still of interest, or it can be a new combination of two or more not-so-new ideas, for example, "Mentor Types and Life Cycles" (Darling, 1984); or perhaps a new slant such as "Elderly Residents: Perceptions of Nurses' Comforting Touch" (Moore & Gilbert, 1995).

Short Manuscripts

Sometimes you may have a short manuscript that is more extensive than a letter to the editor, but not substantive enough for a major article. You might try writing for departments, as mentioned earlier, or write a short-short story. Check which journals published these and use this avenue "for that strongly held conviction of the writer or that urgent message she'd like to convey; for a new perspective on a long-standing situation or a suggestion for an innovative professional direction" (Lewis, 1976, p. 353).

Writing a "shorty survey" is another possibility.

A shorty survey presents a scattered overview of a vast subject. Just as a land surveyor hammers a stake every few hundred feet on a massive tract of land, so the shorty survey alights only on a subject's high points. But it attempts to align high points along a specific, and often seemingly unrelated, theme. A shorty survey looks at a broad subject and picks out some things that can relate to a certain twist (Bryan, 1984, p. 29).

The following list indicates average word counts for several types of writing (Polking, 1983):

Types of Writing	*Words*
Short-short story	500–2,000
Short story	2,500–5,000
Nonfiction book	20,000–200,000

Although the journal article is similar to the short story in length, editors generally have a preferred article length. Do not forget to look for short-short story department opportunities.

NONHEALTH CARE MARKETS

Nurses can also consider other markets for their ideas. When nurses write articles about nursing and health care for nonnursing publications, the results are twofold. First, the image of nurses as health care educators is enhanced. Second, the public benefits from hearing about health care from health professionals.

Friendly Exchange, a quarterly magazine for policyholders of Farmers Insurance Group of Companies occasionally publishes articles pertaining to health and safety. One nurse wrote an article on cochlear implants that was read by a parent whose child later benefited form her newly gained knowledge.

Carol Amen, a nurse who was a prolific writer and writing instructor, wrote the story on which the feature film *Testament* was based. She said,

The biggest service a nurse who is also a writer could do in a professional journal or popular magazine is to talk in everyday, ordinary language, not using 'in' terms or medical jargon. . . . Although I haven't written strictly for nursing journals, the fact that I am a nurse has always influenced all my work—both fiction and nonfiction. Whether health or nursing is mentioned in my stories, I am the person I am partly because of my nursing background. I'm proud that I'm a nurse (Carol Amen, personal communication, January 1984).

SELECTING TARGET JOURNALS

The most important step in getting your article published is to choose the appropriate journal. As you search the literature for the best market for your manuscript, begin to fill in the Target Journal Market Analysis Form (Figure 4.1). Find articles that are similar in concept to the manuscript you want to write. Analyze these articles for theme and audience, style and tone, structure and organization, illustration materials, and personal appeal. Complete the Target Market Analysis form for each journal in which you find an article that is similar to the manuscript you want to write. Try to find three possible markets.

An *Author's Guide to Nursing Journals*, edited by Susan Slaninka (1994), provides useful information about more than 60 nursing journals. This book includes the journal's affiliation, editorial focus or aim, frequency of publication, publisher, manuscript submission information, cover sheet data, required format, acceptance and review, publication length of time, and reprint policy.

We list reference books that will help you select appropriate journals for your articles in Table 4.1. In addition, Appendix 3 lists over 100 nursing and health care publications.

Target Journal Selection and Tracking Form

We developed two tools to help you select target journals and to keep track of responses from editors. Using the Target Journal Market Analysis Form (Figure 4.1) you can better understand the journals. After you have analyzed several possible target journals, look at the possible target journals you have listed on your Writing Plan. Are these still your best choices?

Using the Target Journal Selection and Tracking Form (Figure 4.2), you can look for more markets for your article. Fill in your topic (Column One), then think of two or three general markets to pursue; for example, general nursing journals, educational journals, and clinical nursing specialty journals. Perhaps one category might be to pursue a nonnursing market to reslant your material for a children's or women's magazine or a psychology or medical journal. Write your choices into Column Two—journal markets.

Table 4.1. Reference Books for Selecting Target Journals

Cumulative Index to Nursing and Allied Health Literature (CINAHL)
De Launa Lockwood, ed.
P.O. Box 871
Glendale, CA 91209

A Guide to Writing and Publishing in the Social and Behavioral Sciences
Robert E. Krieger Publishing Company
P.O. Box 9542
Melbourne, FL 32902-9542

International Nursing Index
American Journal of Nursing Company
555 W. 57th St.
New York, New York 10019

Standard Periodical Directory
Oxbridge Communications, Inc.
183 Madison Avenue
New York, NY 10016

Ulrich's International Periodicals Directory
R.R. Bowker
121 Chanlon Road
New Providence, NJ 07974

Writer's Market
Writer's Digest Books
(Annual)
9933 Alliance Road
Cincinnati, Ohio 45242

For each market, select at least three target journals using your journal analyses to guide your selection. You may decide to write for only one market or to have more than three target journals for a market. This form is not to restrict your choices, but rather to facilitate your generating nine targeted journals from one topic. These will be the journals to whom you will inquire about their interest in your manuscript.

As you select target publications, do not feel that you must submit your manuscript only to the most prestigious journal:

Submitting a paper to the most prestigious journal in your field also raises the risk that the paper will not be accepted and that you will have lost weeks, and

Selection

Article Topic	Journal Markets	Target Journals	Working Title

Tracking

Editor/Address	Date of Contact	Editor's Response	Planned Action	Comments

Figure 4.2 Target Journal Selection and Tracking Form (© 1995, Dowdney & Sheridan).

sometimes months, the journal needed to process the paper, sometimes with peer review, before rejecting it. High-prestige journals also have high rejection rates. Because they receive 1,000 to 4,000 manuscripts per year and can publish only a small fraction of these papers, their rejection rates run as high as 90% (Huth, 1982, p. 8).

The Target Journal Selection and Tracking Form (Figure 4.2) will also be your record of journal editor communications. For each target journal, you can complete the editor's name, address, date and type of contact, editor's responses, and follow-up. You will be able to complete the tracking side of this form more easily after you read Chapter Seven, which discusses types of contact with editors. A caution at this point is to not submit your manuscript to more than one editor at a time.

Reconsider your working title. Does it match the type of titles the target journal uses? Remember, the working title is simply your topic stated as a question or descriptive title. Although it may not be a formal title, it will help you focus your query toward a specific audience and journal theme and style. Look at your Writing Plan. Do any of your working titles fit your target journal? Also review your completed Target Journal Analysis Forms and a copy of the target journal's index to create the working title. If you are writing about how the setting in which nurses work affects their work, your title might be "Work Environments Can Enhance Nursing Productivity." If you want to include the effect of the setting on patients, you may have a working title of "The Work Setting Affects the Staff and the Patients." You also might phrase it as a question:"How does the work setting affect staff and patients?" If you know how to measure the effect on staff and patients, then you could change your working title to "The tools That Tell You What Effect Your Work Setting is Having on Your Staff and Patients." This is a working title that could be tightened (fewer words) to your final title.

Make the title as informative and straightforward as possible. You can use a declarative statement or a question, but it should begin with a word or term that represents the most important aspect of the article. Avoid using hyphenated terms because computer search programs may not detect elements of hyphenated terms. Change terms with possessive forms (such as Crohn's disease) to nonpossessive forms (Crohn disease). Use standard rather than nonstandard terms (Council of Biology Editors [CBE], 1994).

After you gather more information on your topic (Chapter Five) and organize the content (Chapter Six), you may evolve to a title such as Porter and Watson did when they wrote "Environment: The Healing Difference." The highlighted caption with this article reads: "The right tools can tell you how well your environment is working for staff and patients alike" (Porter & Watson, 1985, p. 19).

Place your working titles on the Target Journal Selection and Tracking Form. Now you are ready to gather information for the content of your article.

EXERCISES

1. Complete several Target Journal Market Analysis Forms.
2. Complete the selection section of the Target Journal Selection and Tracking Form.

REFERENCES

Andrews, A. C. (1984). Student of nursing . . . student of life. *Imprint, 13*(4), 48.

Bryan, J. (1984, August). Short and, therefore, sweet. *Writer's Digest, 29.*

Council of Biology Editors [CBE]. (1994). *Scientific style and format.* New York: Cambridge University Press.

Cumulative index to nursing and allied health literature. [CINAHL]. (1994). D. Lockwood (Ed.). P. O. Box 871, Glendale, CA 91209.

D'Aquila, N. W., Habegger, D., & Willwreth, E. J. (1994). Converting a QA program to CQI. *Nursing Management, 25*(10), 68–71.

Darling, L. A. W. (1984, November 14). Mentor types and life cycles. *Journal of Nursing Administration, 11,* 43–44.

Dowdney, D. L., & Sheridan, D. R. (1984). *Survey of nursing and health care journal editors.* Unpublished work.

Downs, F. S. (1985). News from the fourth estate. *Nursing Research, 34*(1), 3.

Dumas, M. A. S. (1995). Clinical snapshot: Intermittent claudication. *American Journal of Nursing, 36*(12), 34–35.

Fetzer-Fowler, S. (1984, June). The future of the Baylor plan. *Focus on Critical Care, 11*(3), 53–59.

Fielden, J. S. (1982, May–June). What do you mean you don't like my style? *Harvard Business Review, 138.*

Green, E. (1994). When must indicators be used? *Nursing Quality Connection, 3*(6), 2, 12.

Huth, E. J. (1982). *How to write and publish papers in the medical sciences.* Philadelphia: ISI Press.

International nursing index. New York: American Journal of Nursing Company.

Johnsen, N. M., & Gaspard, M. E. (1985). Theoretical foundations of a prepared sibling class. *Journal of Obstetric, Gynecologic & Neonatal Nursing, 14*(3), 237–242.

Kelly, L. S. (1985). Get one you can control. *Nursing Outlook, 33*(1), 15.

Katz, J. R., & Clemons, P. (1995). Surviving a merger. *Nursing 95, 25*(12), 40–41.

Kim, M. J. (1994). Peer review: When enough is enough. *Image, 26*(4), 257.

Lewis, E. P. (1976). Sounding board. *Nursing Outlook, 24*(6), 353.

Messer, S. S. (1984, March–April). PKU: A mother's perspective. *Pediatric Nursing, 11*(2), 121–123.

Minnick, A., Roberts, M. J., Young, W. B., Kleinpell, R. M., & Micek, W. (1995). An analysis of posthospitalization telephone survey data. *Nursing Research, 44*(6), 371–375.

Moore, J. R., & Gilbert, D. A. (1995). Elderly residents: Perceptions of nurses' comforting touch. *Journal of Gerontological Nursing, 21*(1), 6–13.

Morgan, J. (1984, June). Nutritional assessment of critically ill patients. *Focus on Critical Care, 11*(3), 28–34.

Neubs, H. P. (1994). Sexual harassment: A concern for nursing administrators. *Journal of Nursing Administration, 24*(5), 47–52.

Nursing 95. (1995). Writer's guidelines for *Nursing 95.* [On-line]. Available: Guidelines, 73751, 42.

O'Connor, K. S. (1993). Trailbreaking: Planning for new nursing roles in managed care: Information, innovation, and curriculum. *Aspen Advisor, 8*(12), 1, 3.

Polking, K. (Ed.). (1983). *Writer's encyclopedia.* Cincinnati: Writer's Digest.

Porter, R., & Watson, P. (1985). Environment: The healing difference. *Journal of Nursing Administration, 16*(6), 19.

Rosenberg, H., & Lah, M. I. (1985). Tackling writer's block. *Journal of Nursing Administration, 15*(5), 40.

Rudy, E. B. (1984, June). A view of health care in the USSR. *Focus on Critical Care, 11*(3), 20–27.

Sheridan, D. R. (1983). The health care industry in the marketplace: Implications for nursing. *Journal of Nursing Administration, 13*(9), 36–40.

Slaninka, S. C. (1994). *An author's guide to nursing journals.* King of Prussia, PA: Health Management Publications, Inc.

Strunk, W., Jr., & White, E. B. (1979). *The elements of style.* New York: Macmillan.

Tornquist, E. M. (1983). Strategies for publishing research. *Nursing Outlook, 31*(3), 186.

Wade, G. H. (1995). Is research in the practice setting feasible? *Journal of Continuing Education in Nursing, 26*(6), 253–256.

Weed, R. (1995). A sample of practical technology for the case manager. *The Case Manager, 6*(5), 66–74.

Woods, J. R. (1984, June). Death on a daily basis. *Focus on Critical Care, 11*(3), 50–51.

5

Gather Information

Gathering information is the next step in the writing process. Two major information-gathering methods are searching the literature and interviewing experts. Today computers can help you use both methods. We address searching the literature and interviewing experts in this chapter and offer ideas for using computers and CD-ROMs to help keep you current in nursing, an essential aspect of being a nurse author.

STAYING CURRENT IN NURSING

Reading Nursing Publications

Reading is a key to keeping up-to-date. Although in the past a nurse could read the entire body of periodic nursing literature every month, this is no longer possible. The number of contemporary nursing publications has grown from one, *American Journal of Nursing*, in 1900 to 17 in 1963 to 57 in 1979 (Binger, 1981). By 1984 the *Cumulative Index to Nursing and Allied Health Literature* (CINAHL) listed over 100 contemporary nursing journals in addition to numerous state, alumni, and nonnursing health care publications. The CINAHL now lists over 700 journals in both nursing and allied health fields. The number of journals continues to increase each year. Although you will not be able to read all of them, it is worthwhile to subscribe to and read some of your favorite journals to stay current in your practice area.

You can enlarge your immediate access to more journals if you and your colleagues share journals at work. You may want to circulate journals through your unit or leave them in the room where you and your colleagues take breaks. To encourage reading and comments, staple a comments sheet to the journal's cover. You might begin sharing ideas by writing, "I wish I had read the article on page 8 before we had Mrs. Johnson as a patient—good ideas!"; or, "I disagree with the editorial on page 2 about nurses' career choices. What do you think?"

Participating in a Nursing Journal Club

Another way to stay current is to initiate and participate in a nursing journal club in your work setting. There are many ways for journal clubs to function. Begin with a planning meeting to determine the best time and place to meet. Then use brainstorming techniques to prepare a list of topic areas; rotate responsibility by having one or two nurses comment on articles they select. Other participants can join in the discussion and ask questions, and everyone can complete references providing future access to this data for writing articles.

Another format for journal clubs is to select an article that all participants read, and rotate the responsibility for leading the discussion. Prepared questions focus the discussion. It is especially useful to discuss "How can we use the information in our setting?" and "Does this discussion stimulate any article ideas?"

Your journal club may also become a source of a co-authored article on an unanswered question, difference of opinion, or unique approach to dealing with a similar problem or meeting a similar need. You may want to challenge some part of the article, take the author's ideas one step further, or apply the author's suggestions to your specialty setting. Besides staying current, your discussion may lead to the synergistic development of new article ideas. A word of caution—do not try to write an article as a large group. If you meet regularly, many article ideas will result, and you can work in pairs to develop these ideas into query letters. Participating in an online journal club is another way to keep pace with other professionals through peer-reviewed journal articles. Members of the American Medical Association can receive CME credits as they participate in lively journal discussion groups as part of the JAMA Journal Club.

Scanning the Nursing Indices

In your efforts to keep up-to-date, scan nursing indices regularly. This way even if you do not have time to read an entire journal, you can read the index and skim articles. You will be surprised at how much you will remember, and your awareness of current issues in the nursing literature will expand amazingly.

If you do not subscribe, but have access to a library with nursing journals, stop at the library once a month on the way to or from work. Scan the indices—read several articles or copy a few for bedtime reading. Watch for articles related to topics on your idea list. Regular reading of journal articles is one of the best ways to prepare yourself as a nurse writer. It is valuable to read extensively and widely within and beyond nursing and health care.

CONDUCTING THE LIBRARY SEARCH

As you begin your library search, you will be preparing an inventory of all promising printed sources. Therefore, bring two sizes of index cards with you, 3" x 5" and 4" x 6". Use the 3" x 5" cards to create a bibliography ("bib") card for each journal, magazine, book, pamphlet, or online source that you use.

Your bib card will include the full name of each author or editor, the complete title of each publication or online source, and the publication details. Place the author's last name at the top so that you can file the cards alphabetically. Include the author's first name because some journals, such as the *Journal of Nursing Administration*, require first names in the reference lists. On the next line, place the publication's date. Follow with the full title and publication details, including the number or description of the edition, the volume and issue numbers, the place of publication, and the publisher's name. Conclude with specific page numbers. Add a notation about where you found the book or journal, particularly if you use various libraries. This note will help you the next time you need to locate the publication. Figure 5.1 is an example of a "bib card."

If you tend to forget a fact or two when you jot down references, you can make copies of the bibliography card with guidelines (Figure 5.2) and take these with you to the library to remind yourself of the information you need for each reference citation.

Use the 4" x 6" index cards for taking notes on the content in the publications. The following are practical tips on preparing your note cards:

- Write only one idea on each card.
- Do not make cryptic notes that will be difficult to decipher later.
- Prepare a key for any symbols you use.
- Organize the notes into a system according to how you will use the data.
- Place quotation marks around all direct quotations.
- Paraphrase information to keep the essential meaning of the original information.

Sheridan, Donna Richards
Dowdney, Donna Lee
1996
How to Write and Publish Articles in Nursing
2nd edition
New York: Springer
p. 93

Palo Alto City Library

Figure 5.1. Bibliography "bib" card.

Author
Date
Title of Publication
Title of Article or Chapter
Edition
Publisher
Address
Volume
Issue
Pages
Library Used

Figure 5.2. Bibliography card form with guidelines.

You can put these index cards into your individual idea files until you are ready to write, or you can file them alphabetically by topic. An index card for note-taking should include the topic as well as the author's name. These information cards cross-reference with the bib cards by author, yet allow you to sort information by topic when you organize your article. You can, for a less detailed search, use the backs of bib cards for notes. However, if you put more than one topic on a card, it will be difficult to use your cards later when you organize your article.

Leslie H. Nicholl (1993, pp. 13–14) observed that "Just as using paper indexes is no longer sufficient for doing a literature search, index cards no longer make the grade as a way to organize a bibliography." The article, "Managing Bibliographic Information," stated that by using computer-based strategies to retrieve literature resources "suddenly you are overwhelmed with information." Nicholl then reviewed two computer software programs that manage databases by organizing references and creating bibliographies: "As information is continually expanding at an alarming rate, it is important to have easy-to-use, dependable methods to manage the chaos." The software programs offer a computer-based alternative to index cards.

Another way to gather information is to photocopy relevant articles. After you read and highlight major points of articles on any topic in your file, place the copies in your idea file. When the idea file bulges, split your files into individual new file folders on specific topics. These become reference files for your individual articles—one file per article.

Your reading of current articles and reviewing of your article files will help you write your query letter to editors (Chapter 7 describes the query letter.) You will also have a ready source of ideas for beginning to write your article, an inservice education program, a lecture, speech, or literature search.

Searching the Literature

Searing the literature helps you find out what is already known about your topic. Searching also expands your understanding of topics and helps you fit them into a broader context. Literature searches will increase your efficiency and effectiveness in writing. Even if you are current in your specialty, you will usually need to review the nursing literature before you write a manuscript.

"Searching" Versus "Researching"

The word *research* implies that you are using the research method to solve problems. In contrast, *searching* means to look at or examine carefully; to inquire, investigate; to conduct an examination or investigation. What you are usually doing in the library is searching, not researching.

Using Special Libraries

To find special libraries, consult the *American Library Directory*, published by the R. R. Bowker Company. The 1994–1995 edition lists 32,625 libraries in the United States and 4,001 libraries in Canada. In the category of special libraries, this reference book includes 2,443 medical libraries in the United States and 276 medical libraries in Canada. It arranges listings geographically by state or province and city. Then it gives specific information about particular libraries.

For example, to find out about the Lane Medical Library at Stanford University Medical Center, you would use Volume 1 of the *American Library Directory, Libraries in the United States*. Then find "California" and "Stanford" in the library listings. The letter "M" in the margin for "Medical" draws your attention to Lane Medical Library. It then shows the addresses, telephone numbers, e-mail addresses, fax numbers, names of key librarians, book holdings, special collections, automation information (number and types of computers available), online catalog information, and participation in various library cooperatives.

Eight Regional Medical Libraries of the National Library of Medicine are located throughout the United States. See Table 5.1 for their addresses and telephone and fax numbers.

Universities and colleges often have excellent libraries and may allow nonstudents to use them. Another information source is a hospital library. Although hospital libraries may be small, they are part of a national network that the National Library of Medicine (NLM) sponsors.

Using Library Resources

Take your topic file, 3" x 5" and 4" x 6" index cards, coins for the photocopy machines, several pencils, and a pad of paper with you to the library. You may also want to bring a magnifying glass to read small print! Begin your search by listing all the terms related to your topic.

Next, find the two most comprehensive and authoritative indices for locating nursing journals: *Cumulative Index to Nursing and Allied Health Literature* (CINAHL) and *The International Nursing Index* (INI). The *Cumulative Index to Nursing and Allied Health Literature* indexes nursing, allied health, and health-related journals for inclusion in its five bimonthly issues and yearly cumulative bound volume. It also indexes pertinent articles from biomedical journals indexed in *Index Medicus*, as well as relevant material from popular journals. This publication is the only index to nursing periodicals from 1960 to 1965. It indexes the majority of nursing periodicals published in English. In addition, it indexes publications of the National League for Nursing, the American Nurses' Association, and, since 1972, the state nursing associations.

Since 1977 CINAHL has extended its coverage to include the periodical literature of cardiopulmonary technology, emergency services, health education, health science librarianship, medical and laboratory technology, the medical assistant, medical records, occupational therapy, physical therapy and rehabilitation, radiologic technology, respiratory therapy, and social service in health care.

CINAHL is available online as well as on CD-ROM (Compact Disk Read-Only Memory). CD-ROM technology packages entire volumes of ref-

Table 5.1. Regional Medical Libraries

Regional Medical Library	Address	Phone/Fax
Middle Atlantic	New York Academy of Medicine 2 E. 103rd St. New York, NY 10029	Ph: (212) 876-8763 Fax: (212) 534-7042
Southeastern/Atlantic	University of Maryland at Baltimore Health Sciences Library 111 S. Greene St. Baltimore, MD 21201-1583	Ph: (410) 706-2855 Fax: (410) 706-0099
Greater Midwest	University of Illinois at Chicago Library of the Health Sciences P.O. Box 7509 Chicago, IL 60680	Ph: (312) 996-2464 Fax: (312) 996-2226

Midcontinental	University of Nebraska
	  Medical Center
	Leon S. McGoogan
	  Library of Medicine
	600 S. 42nd St.
	Omaha, NB 68198-6706
		Ph: (402) 559-4326
		
		Fax: (402) 559-5482

South Central	Houston Academy of Medicine Texas Medical Center Library 1133 M.D. Anderson Blvd. Houston, TX 77030	Ph: (713) 790-7053 Fax: (713) 790-7030
Pacific Northwest	University of Washington Health Center Library, SB-55 Seattle, WA 98195	Ph: (206) 543-8262 Fax: (206) 543-2469

Pacific Southwest	University of California,
	  Los Angeles
	Louise Darling
	  Biomedical Library
	10833 Le Conte Ave.
	Los Angeles, CA 90024-1798
		Ph: (310) 825-1200
		
		Fax: (310) 825-5389

New England	University of Connecticut
	  Health Center
	Lyman Maynard Stowe Library,
	  ASB-3
	263 Farmington Ave.
	Farmington, CT 06030-5370
		Ph: (203) 679-4500
		
		Fax: (203) 679-1305

Eight Regional Medical Libraries are responsible for specific geographic areas of the National Network of Libraries of Medicine. The toll-free telephone number for all Regional Medical Libraries is 1-800-338-7657 (or 1-800-338-RMLS).

erence sources on single read-only disks. One CINAHL CD-ROM holds all the data found in print indexes dating back to 1983. Thus, you can search many years' information at one time, rather than searching one year at a time by using printed volumes.

Another CD-ROM resource of interest to nurses is MEDLINE (MEDical Literature Analysis and Retrieval System On-Line). MEDLINE became operational in 1971. It contains over 7 million journal articles dating back to 1966. Abstracts are available for 60% of references from 1975 to the present. MEDLINE is produced by the U.S. National Library of Medicine and is one of the major sources for biomedical literature materials. It corresponds to three print indexes: *Index Medicus,* the *International Nursing Index,* and the *Index to Dental Literature.* A benefit of using the CD-ROM version of MEDLINE is to practice using various search strategies without having to consider the cost of connect time.

Bonnie Westra and Karen Larsen (1994) point out that by using CD-ROM, you can limit your search in ways that the print version does not offer. You can specify the type of publication you want, such as articles or books, and you can limit your search to a specific author, certain publication years, age groups, or practice settings. You can also specify that you need research articles, case studies, or care plans.

The International Nursing Index (INI), which exclusively indexes nursing publications, has been published quarterly in cooperation with the National Library of Medicine since 1966. It is also the basis for the nursing material in MEDLINE. INI indexes over 250 nursing periodicals as well as all nursing articles in the nonnursing journals currently indexed in *Index Medicus.* INI has subject and name sections and includes lists of nursing periodicals and serials indexed, current nursing publications of organizations and agencies, and books for or by nurses. It also lists doctoral dissertations under the name of the institutions in which they were written. The INI provides comprehensive coverage of the nursing literature in all languages. *The International Nursing Index* also contains the *Nursing Thesaurus.* The *Nursing Thesaurus* gives commonly used nursing terms as cross-references to the subject headings used in INI.

The *Hospital Literature Index* is prepared quarterly, with annual cumulations. The U.S. National Library of Medicine compiles *Index Medicus* monthly. This is the foremost index in medicine; professionals in related fields commonly use it. An annual *Cumulated Index Medicus* contains subject and author indexes to articles selected from thousands of biomedical journals. It includes a bibliography of medical reviews.

Using the latest copy of these indexes, look up all the terms on your list and place markers in each page. One term may suggest another to you. If this happens, add the new term to your list for inclusion in your investigation. Photocopy relevant pages of the indexes. Repeat this procedure for the last 3 years and for current monthly editions. Another source of information about articles related to your topic is the reference lists or bibliographies following relevant articles you have already located.

Now, rank the articles as to how closely they relate to your topic. Give each article a priority number in the margin of the copied index page:

1. *High priority:* You absolutely must have the article. It looks suspiciously like the one you are about to write, or it contains your topic.
2. *Medium priority:* You will find the article desirable because it is closely related to your topic.
3. *Low priority:* You may find the article useful, but it is not essential for your topic.

Then, begin with the high and medium priorities. Look for these articles in the stacks, or order them through an interlibrary loan. If you do not find the article you need, search more broadly. Consider your library search as similar to finding pieces of a puzzle. Although you may not find the specific piece you are looking for to fit into the puzzle, you will get a better understanding of your project.

After you find the journals, review the top-priority articles. If they are relevant to your topic, photocopy them or order reprints from the publishers. Several currently published authors indicated that they use the photocopy method because it increases efficiency and decreases errors. As an alternative to photocopying, you may prefer to read the article in the library and use your bib cards and note cards. If you do this, remember to write a complete citation (see Figure 5.2) so that you can retrieve the article to cite the reference in your manuscript.

This preliminary search may be sufficient for preparing your entire article, depending on the topic and type of article. Read the photocopied articles, marking or highlighting relevant points—both those that agree with and those that differ from your perspective. Read everything directly related to the topic before you begin to write.

Do not try to simply string quotations together for an article. Use others' thoughts as beginning points or to show supporting or contrasting perspectives. You need to spend time thinking about your topic in relation to what is in the nursing literature. No amount of literature review can replace thinking and integrating your ideas into your manuscript.

Performing an Online Computer Search

To obtain the most recently published information on a topic, conduct an online database search. Online databases are collections of specialized and related information stored in a computer's memory that you use a computer to search. Many databases are bibliographic and provide abstracts. Typical bibliographic databases are composed of over 1 million records. Each record is made up of a series of fields, each representing one piece of information that describes one particular aspect of a document. For example, in the "source" field are journal name, volume, source number, pagination, and publication date. Some databases include full text of the articles referenced.

Computer searches are faster and more complete than manual searches. They search topics by combining qualifying factors to exclude irrelevant material. Computer literature searches have become essential for gathering the most current information. Hundreds of journals and thousands of articles are available to you when you conduct computer searches.

Using computers provides a number of advantages over print searching, according to Kirstin C. Nichols (1994, p. 58):

- The computer can combine concepts, saving hours of time in searches involving a subject with multiple concepts.
- The computerized form of *Index Medicus* (MEDLINE) has more information than the printed form, including authors' abstracts and all the Medical Subject Headings.
- The verification of references by doing a quick online search may be the most time- and cost-effective way to fill in missing information—particularly for unknown or questionable dates. This is because index volumes are issued by year and do not allow author searches. Online searches are the only way to search by article title or by specific words in the title.
- The online search with a personal computer offers the convenience of information retrieval at your desk.

There are several approaches to a computer search. In order to retrieve the data relevant to your topic, a librarian may use more than one approach. Because computer time is charged by the minute, librarians plan the search before accessing the computer database to make the most efficient use of computer time. The librarian will ask you to complete a form containing a description of your topic along with alternate terms from appropriate thesauri and complete citations for one or two related articles. Thus, manual searching precedes a good computer search.

Taking shortcuts can waste time. For example, one computer search performed on "nursing orientation" (that is, orientation to the job) elicited an entire printout on nursing references to "orientation" (and disorientation—to place and person). Good work in advance results in high-quality results.

One approach to the search is to enter at least two terms at a time. For instance, if you are looking for information on writing for nursing publications, select key words such as *writing, publications,* and *nursing.* Such a search produced a citation and an abstract for S. Fondiller's article on "Writing for Publication." The article appeared in the *American Journal of Nursing* in August 1994. The citation appeared with the following abstract: "If you've never written an article before, it can seem like a monumental task. These tips will ease their way." This short abstract gives enough information for searchers to decide if the article is relevant for their projects.

Another approach that librarians may use for searching is to enter the name of the related article from your search form. Then the librarian can query the database to find out what terms were used to reference that article and use those terms for you computer search.

The list of terms you already developed will help in the computer search. Articles close to your topic will also give you access to your topic in the database. Request that a librarian perform a search that will give you a printout of references to books and periodicals, as well as other information sources. We also recommend that you request abstracts whenever possible because abstracts provide more information about the relevance of certain articles—relying on titles alone may be misleading.

In her workshop given at American Medical Writer's Association conferences on *Bibliographic Resources for Medical Communicators,* Joan N. Nilson (1995, p. 37) offers the following online search guidelines:

1. Choose the best database or databases for the search.
2. Use the system or vendor that offers the most appropriate databases at the best price.
3. Always check database documentation before searching an unfamiliar database.
4. Make sure that you know your database system's default for Boolean operators, as execution varies.
5. Know the purpose and motivation of the search, as well as the level of information needed.
6. Create your search strategy before you go online, but remain flexible enough to modify your search strategy if it proves to be inadequate or unproductive.
7. Use cost-effective search techniques.
8. Save all your searches on a computer disk.
9. Develop an online searching style, but know when to try something different.
10. Remember: there is no totally right way to do a search and conversely: there are very few totally wrong ways to do a search!

In conclusion, reference librarians can help you focus your computer search by working with the keywords you select from the *Nursing Thesaurus.* Reference librarians will also help you determine the appropriate number of sources to search and will indicate costs involved of various types of searches.

The National Library of Medicine maintains and operates a computerized, online information system. The Regional Medical Library Network and the National Library of Medicine allows you to gain access to publications not available from local libraries. Nursing, medicine, and health care libraries can request loans from Regional Medical Libraries. Table 5.1 lists the eight Regional Medical Libraries along with their addresses, telephone numbers, and fax numbers.

MEDLINE indexes original journal articles and editorials. Many software vendors provide software to allow access to MEDLINE and other databases. The vendors' services vary in their time of availability, cost structure for online time, and print or download charges, monthly minimum payments, types of acceptable accounts such as charge or deposit accounts, search limits, and compatibility with high-speed modems.

An online information system such as MEDLINE allows you to have direct access to a database and the computer's processing capability. Online terminals are electronically linked to the main computer's memory. To learn what databases are available, consult an index that lists databases such as *Computer Readable Data Bases: A Directory and Data Sourcebook* (Marcaccio, 1991). The 1991 edition covers 6,750 databases. Also, speak with a librarian about newly available databases. Table 5.2 lists selected computer-readable databases of interest to nurses. Nurses may perform searches at their desktops by using simplified versions of selected databases or by using appropriate commercial online services.

Some user-friendly software systems offer access to various databases. PaperChase allows access to MEDLINE Health *STAR, AIDSLINE,* and *CANCERLIT.* DIALOG has a wide list of databases with menu-driven access. Grateful Med allows access to other National Library of Medicine databases, such as AIDSLINE and TOXLINE. Table 5.3 shows contact information for selected online services and software.

Typically, organizations lease databases from publishers through online vendors such as DIALOG or BRS who make the databases available for searching. Over 1,000 online systems are available. Of these systems, over 2,000 database producers feature more than 5,000 databases.

After you or your organization subscribe to one of the database vendors, such as the National Library of Medicine (NLM), you can connect to databases across the nation and around the world by using a modem connected to a computer. To access MEDLINE, the main database of the MEDLARS group, use your pre-arranged user identification and a password.

Commercial information services also provide access to medical and health databases. For example, CompuServe's healthcare and medical services offer a variety of information to consumers and healthcare providers. Its communication features include e-mail, forums, and Internet access. Table 5.4 shows selected examples of online medical and health resources on CompuServe.

The Internet

The Internet is the name for a group of worldwide information resources. The Internet is growing at a rate of 100% per year, based on the number of hosts connected to the Internet. The Internet Society projects that there will be an estimated 120 million hosts worldwide by the turn of the century.

> Libraries are the most visible and numerous resources on the Internet. You can visit college libraries, public and private libraries, national libraries, corporate libraries, scientific libraries, and even virtual libraries with electronic books, all over the world. The U.S. Library of Congress has even developed a virtual library catalog, the L.C. Marvel that you can browse through like any other electronic card catalog. (Eddings, 1994, p. 9)

Once you have your connection to the Internet, you can perform the activities as described in the following section:

- Send and receive electronic mail
- Use Telnet to log onto other computers
- Use the World Wide Web
- Reach resources such as MEDLINE and other databases
- Participate in Usenet, Forums, and Newsgroups
- Use Internet Gophers to browse information

Electronic Mail. Electronic mail (e-mail) is the primary use of the Internet and is the equivalent of postal mail except that it is faster and cheaper. According to William Grant, principal programmer/analyst in the Systems Technology Group of Informix, in 1995, 95 billion e-mail messages were sent in the United States alone, exceeding the total mail sent by the U.S. Postal Service by 10 billion pieces (Grant, 1995, pp. 17–24). By using the Internet, you can use e-mail to contact other Internet subscribers. Sally Squires, a staff writer for the Health section of *The Washington Post*, says "E-mail is one way of contacting sources. You can say, 'I'm trying to reach you.' A colleague did an entire interview via e-mail with someone who was difficult to reach" (Squires, 1966, p. 3). Squires usually conducts e-mail interviews with professors or principal investigators. First, she calls their offices to confirm that they are who they are supposed to be. Then she e-mails them questions. She

Table 5.2. Selected Computer-Readable Databases of Interest to Nurses

Contact Information	Overview	Topics Covered
AVLINE U.S. National Library of Medicine (NLM) MEDLARS Management Section 8600 Rockville Pike, Bethesda, MD 20894 (301) 496-6193	Bibliographic citations to audiovisual material in clinical medicine as catalogued by MEDLARS. Includes motion pictures, videocassettes, slide/cassette, and filmstrip/cassette programs. Covers 1975 to present. Contains over 20,000 records. Updated weekly.	Audiovisual material in clinical medicine, ranging from anatomy to zoology. Input sources are audiovisual materials catalogued at the National Library of Medicine.
MEDLINE U.S. National Library of Medicine (NLM) MEDLARS Management Section 8600 Rockville Pike, Bethesda, MD 20894 (301) 496-6193	Bibliographic citations to the world's journal literature in biomedicine, nursing, dentistry, and related topics. Covers 1966 to the present. Contains over 6,000,000 records. Updated weekly.	Medicine (preclinical and clinical sciences), life sciences and other health-sciences topics. Input sources are 3,900 journals prior to 1981.
CINAHL Nursing & Allied Health Database 1509 Wilson Terrace P.O. Box 871 Glendale, CA 91209-0871 (818) 409-8005	Bibliographic database. Indexes and abstracts articles appearing in more than 300 current English-language nursing journals, publications of the American Nurses' Association and the National League for Nursing, and journals in more than a dozen allied health disciplines. Also includes nursing dissertations and selected articles appearing in 3,200 biomedical journals, 20	Nursing and allied health professions including cardiopulmonary technology, emergency services, health education, health sciences librarianship, medical and laboratory technology, medical assistance, medical records, occupational therapy, physician's assistant, physical therapy and rehabilitation, radiologic technology, respiratory therapy, social service in health

Table 5.2. (*continued*)

Contact Information	Overview	Topics Covered
	journals in health science librarianship, books from approximately 30 healthcare publishers, and education, psychological, management, and popular literature. Covers 1983 to the present with over 85,000 records. Updated monthly.	care, and surgical technology. Input sources are more than 300 nursing journals plus proceedings, professional publications, and government documents. Relevant citations from 3,200 journals indexed in Index Medicus are retrieved from the MEDLARS system for inclusion in the database.
PsycINFO American Psychological Association (APA) Psychological Abstracts Information Services 1400 N. Uhle St. Arlington, VA 22201 (703) 247-7829	Bibliographic database containing citations and nonevaluative summaries of the world's literature dealing with psychology and related fields. Covers 1967 to the present with over 700,000 records. Updated monthly.	All areas of psychology including experimental and developmental, communications, social processes and issues, personality, physical and psychological disorders, professional issues, applied psychology, and educational psychology. Behavioral literature in related fields such as law, business, and medicine. Input sources are more than 1,300 periodicals, technical reports, dissertations, and other sources.
TOXLINE U.S. National Library of Medicine (NLM) Toxicology Information Program (TIP) 8600 Rockville Pike Bethesda, MD 20894 (301) 496-1131	Bibliographic database provides citations to published sources on pharmacological, biochemical, psychological, and toxicological effects of drugs and other chemicals. Covers 1965 to the present. Contains over 2,500,000 references. Updated monthly.	Biological and adverse effects of drugs, human and animal toxicity, pesticides, environmental chemicals and pollutants, food additives, industrial and household chemicals, and radioactive materials.

Based on Marcaccio, 1991.

Table 5.3. Contact Information for Selected Online Services and Software

Services and Software	Address	Telephone
America Online	8619 Westwood Center Dr. Vienna, VA 22182-2285 http://www.aol.com	(800) 827-6364
BRS Information Technologies	Maxwell Online 800 Westpark Dr. McLean, VA 22102	(800) 955-0906
CompuServe Information Service	5000 Arlington Centre Blvd. Columbus, OH 43220 http://www. compuserve.com	(800) 848-8199
DELPHI, General Videotex Corp.	3 Blackstone St. Cambridge, MA 02139	(800) 544-4005
Knight-Ridder Information DIALOG, DIALOGLINK, DIALOG OnDisc, MEDLINE, Knowledge Index, Medical Connection, DIALOG Menus, DIALOG Information Services	3460 Hillview Ave. Palo Alto, CA 94304 http://www.krinfo.com	(800) 3-DIALOG
GRATEFUL MED, National Technical Center, U.S. Dept. of Commerce	5285 Port Royal Road Springfield, VA 22161	(703) 487-4650
MEDLINE, GRATEFUL MED, National Library of Medicine	MEDLARS Management 8600 Rockville Pike Bethesda, MD 20209	(800) 638-8480
MSN The Microsoft Network	One Microsoft Way Redmond, WA 98052-6399	(800) 386-5550
Prodigy	445 Hamilton Ave. White Plains, NY 10601 http://www.prodigy.com	(800) PRODIGY

finds that e-mail is faster than telephone voice mail, and it gets peoples' attention in a different way. She recommends that writers always double-check the e-mail responses to confirm who actually sent them (Squires, 1996).

Telnet. You can also log into other computers, called remote computers. By logging into remote computers, you can search libraries of information around the world and transfer that data back to your own computer. Telnet is an Internet facility that lets you execute commands on remote computers as if you logged in locally. To establish a Telnet connection, you use the name of the computer site you want to access. You must have a valid user name and password for that site, although some Telnet sites allow for guest logins. Guest accounts typically are restricted as to the types of actions users can perform during a Telnet session. Although your Telnet session is actually running software directly on the site's Telnet computer, you will be running a program that prevents you from accessing the general capabilities of that computer.

Once you connect to a Telnet site, you will often see a menu-driven system under the control of the Telnet site. The menu guides you through the actions you may perform at that site. Another common use of Telnet is for users to log into their computers from remote locations. In this case, you would enter your user name and password and have the same user privileges you would have when logged in without using Telnet.

The World Wide Web: The internet unleashed. The World Wide Web is part of the Internet and consists of a huge collection of documents stored on computers around the world. A web page is a document on the World Wide Web that could include text, pictures, sound, or movies. Web sites are colleges, government agencies, or companies that store web pages. Each web page has a unique address called the Uniform Resource Locator (URL). All Web page URLs start with "http." As you surf the Web, you can select interesting items on pages to jump to other pages. Then you can store the new Web page on the same computer or on a computer across the city, country, or world. Jumping from one Web page to another lets you browse through a vast amount of information without needing to know where the information is stored. (MaranGraphics, 1996).

No innovation in recent history has been so well received and widely implemented as the World Wide Web ('Web'). A framework of previous and new innovations, the Web is quickly redefining the way business, research and communications are conducted. On a par with the telephone, radio, and television, the Web is a communications evolution of revolutionary proportions (Grant, 1995, pp. 17–24).

Table 5.4. Selected Online Medical and Health Resources on CompuServe

Type of Resource	Description of Online Resource
Research Databases Basic Services (GO DRUGS)	*Consumer Reports* Complete Drug Reference as compiled by the U.S. Pharmacopeia. General information about the correct use of medicine. Individual entries on a variety of drugs. Search by generic or brand name.
Research Databases Basic Services (GO HNT)	HealthNet provides useful general information for consumers. Concise reference library of health, medical, and sports medicine. Search by disease, symptoms, drugs, surgeries or tests.
Research Databases Basic Services (GO AIDSNEWS)	AIDS News Clips lists news reports on AIDS supplied by the Associated Press, Reuters, United Press International, and *The Washington Post*. Updated throughout the day.
Research Databases Extended Services (GO HANDICAPPED)	Handicapped Users' Database gives information on software, hardware, organizations, news, research and development as well as a reference library.
Research Databases Extended Services (GO HSX)	Human Sexuality Databank provides general information on urology, gynecology, psychiatry, and other fields of sexual medicine and therapy. Searchable databank, support groups, and forums.
Research Databases Extended Services (GO NORD)	Rare Disease Database is sponsored by the National Organization for Rare Disorders. Offers information on rare diseases including symptoms, causes, standard and investigational therapies, and other resources.
Research Databases Extended Services with Surcharges (GO CCMLAIDS)	CCML AIDS provides full-text AIDS-related articles from the Comprehensive Core Medical Library. It includes resources from medical reference books, textbooks, and general medical journals.

Table 5.4. (*continued*)

Type of Resource	Description of Online Resource
Research Databases Extended Services with Surcharges (GO HLTDB)	Health Database Plus is designed for consumers. It contains articles from consumer and professional publications on topics related to health, fitness, nutrition, and healthcare politics.
Research Databases Extended Services with Surcharges (GO IQMEDICINE)	Quest Medical InfoCenter provides comprehensive access to medical, pharmaceutical, and allied health databases including AIDS Weekly, Allied and Alternative Medicine, Cancer Research Weekly, Combined Health Information Database and MEDLINE.
Research Databases Extended Services with Surcharges (GO KI)	Knowledge Index offers weekend and evening access only to medical and pharmaceutical databases at reduced rates. Databases include CancerLit, International Pharmaceutical Abstracts, Merck Index Online, PsychINFO, Mental Health Abstracts, and more.
Research Databases Extended Services with Surcharges (GO PAPERCHASE)	PaperChase offers menu-driven access to MEDLINE. It contains more than 8 million references to articles from 4,000 journals.
Research Databases Extended Services with Surcharges (GO PSYCIN)	PsychINFO offers abstracts on psychology and behavior sciences. Covers applied, developmental, general and experimental psychology.

Cyberlibrarian Cynthia N. James-Catalano shared an example of places to find information about breast cancer in her article, "The Good Fight." She wrote:

> There are many places on the Internet to obtain information about this disease that affects one woman in nine. On the Web at http://www.med.stanford.edu/CBHP/ you'll find the Community Breast Health Project, whose mission is to improve the lives of those touched by breast cancer. It is a patient-driven resource and has pages of medical information that can make the procedures that cancer patients face less confusing. There are also lists of events and organizations that can help patients and their families.
>
> At the site you'll find the personal account of Jenilu Schoolman, who has been optimistically fighting the disease since she was told she would die of it eight years ago. At the end of her story, you are invited to write to her and join a breast cancer discussion group. (You can subscribe to the discussion group by sending e-mail to listserv@morgan.ucs.mun.ca with subscribe breastcancer in the message body.) (James-Catalano, 1995, p. 34)

The article also shares the address of Avon's Breast Cancer Awareness Crusade page at http://www.pmedia.com/Avon/avon.html. This offers frequently asked questions, facts, and a list of toll-free numbers for obtaining further help and information. It also contains a glossary of terms and a special section on mammograms. In addition, the article mentions the Breast Cancer Information Clearinghouse at http://nysernet.org/bcic/.

The Web's goal is to provide a uniform way to access hypermedia documents from any location on the Internet. Through the development of graphical user interface (GUI) browsers, such as Mosaic or Netscape's Navigator, users possess a seamless browser interface that hides most of the Internet's complexity.

In this article "Electric Texts," Steve O'Keefe wrote about hypertextbooks, which are digital documents that are like having a tutor built into every book. He cites an example of the Virtual Hospital:

> Almost no one has made more use of multimedia hypertextbooks than the Virtual Hospital. Located at the University of Iowa College of Medicine, you'll find its hypermedia library at http:///vh.radiology.uiowa.edu/Providers/Textbooks/Multimedia Textbooks.html.
>
> The Virtual Hospital offers hypertextbooks on such subjects as lung anatomy, pulmonary embolus, joint fluoroscopy, and gastrointestinal nuclear medicine. The presentations are heavily illustrated and fully hyperlinked to encyclopedias and other help resources. The multimedia exhibits include not only still photos, but MPEG movies and sound files.

Other resources available at the Virtual Hospital include teaching files, clinical guidelines, and assorted professional publications (O'Keefe, 1995, p. 58).

Table 5.5 shows selected World Wide Web sites of interest to nurses and healthcare providers.

MEDLINE.   MEDLINE is the National Library of Medicine (NLM) database. You can reach MEDLINE if you have an account and Internet access. The MEDLINE database contains millions of articles from over 4,000 medical journals and publications. "You can find complete bibliographic information, such as title, author, publication, date of publication, keywords, and much more. MEDLINE pulls this data together, allowing researchers to look in just one place" (Eddings, 1994, p. 43).

Usenet, Forums, and Newsgroups on the Internet

Usenet (contraction of "User's Network") is a system of discussion groups in which individual articles are distributed throughout the world. After e-mail, Usenet is the second most popular application of the Internet. Usenet consists of thousands of computers that receive Network News organized into newsgroups. Participating in forums or newsgroups is another way to gather and share information with other nurses and health care professionals. Usenet is a global network and community. Usenet works on a cooperative basis by storing articles and then forwarding them from Usenet computer to computer.

Nurses have a special area on USENET in which to share ideas, anecdotes, and technical information on all aspects of nursing. *The Internet Yellow Pages* (1995) lists three newsgroups for nurses:

alt.npractitioners
bit.listerv.snurse-1
sci.med.nursing

Anne Hart, a medical journalist, posed the following question on the newsgroup alt.support.menopause. "Is anyone else using a high soy and vegetarian diet, the herb black cohosh, and natural, yam-derived, progesterone cream for menopause—to help prevent bone loss—instead of the usual estrogen and progestin? If so, what are your comments and experiences?" She wrote that the replies she received were practical, useful, and factual. Her correspondents provided medical references, titles, journal articles, book bibliographies, as well as personal experiences and encouragement (Hart, 1996, p. 42).

Table 5.5. Selected World Wide Web Sites for Healthcare Providers

---

American Heart Association
http://www.amhrt.org

Anesthesiology & Surgery Center
http://www-sci.lib.uci.edu/HSG/MedicalSurgery.html

Cancer Related Links
http://dialin.ind.net/~rmarriag/rcancer.html

Centers for Disease Control and Prevention
http://www.cdc.gov

Global Health Network
http://info.pitt.edu/HOME/GHNet/GHNet.html

Health Letter on the CDC
http://ip.holonet.net/homepage/1d.htm

Health on the Internet Newsletter
http://www.pavilion.co.uk/daccess/D-Access/newsletters/HOT.html

Hospital Web
http://demOmac.mgh.harvard.edu/hospitalweb.html

HyperDOC
http://www.nlm.nih.gov

LifeNet
http://www.awinc.com/partners/bc/compass/lifenet/lifenet.htm

The Mayo Clinic
http://www.mayo.edu

National Institutes of Health
http://www.nih.gov

Virtual Hospital
http://vh-radiology-uiowa.edu

Women's Health Hot Line Newsletter
http://www.soft-design.com/softinfo/womens-health.html

Internet gophers.   Internet "Gophers" provide a series of menus from which you can browse information, including that provided by other Internet resources. The Nightingale gopher and mailing list include nursing, research, practice, education, and nursing publications; professional nursing communications; and other nursing resources.

CompuServe also provides two forums that can help you use CompuServe's Internet services. The Internet New Users Forum (GO INET-NEWUSER) provides help and support in using CompuServe's Internet services. In this forum, you will find information on using CompuServe Mail to send e-mail to Internet addresses, on accessing the USENET newsgroups, etc. The Internet New Users Forum is the place to go for this kind of basic "How do It. . ." support. See Table 5.6 for forums of interest to nurses.

The Internet Resources Forum (GO INETRESOURCES) contains extensive information about the resources accessible through the Internet. Much like the reference desk of a public library, the Internet Resources Forum contains the latest news and information about the vast range of information resources available on the Internet. Although primarily valuable to experienced users of the Internet, the Internet Resources Forum is also the place for newcomers to learn more specific information on the Internet and to answer the "Where can I find . . ." questions.

Another online source of information for nurses is *The On-Line Journal of Knowledge Synthesis for Nursing*. This journal offers timely, synthesized knowledge to guide nursing practice and research. It provides a critical review of research pertinent to clinical practice and research situations that nurses can access and use immediately. The journal helps nurses stay abreast of the vast amount of published scientific information. You can access this journal via the Internet using Guidon 2.0. Your work station must have a direct TCP/IP connection to the Internet, either via an installed ethernet or token ring board, or via dial access to a host computer supporting the Serial-Line Interface Protocol (SLIP).

Subscribers can search articles online and review, download, and print relevant information in whole or part. Readers can electronically search by subject, title, author, keyword, date, phrase, or combination of words. In a single search, readers can cover the entire collection of *Knowledge Synthesis for Nursing* articles.

The Virginia Henderson International Nursing Library is now available online. This electronic library is a computerized collection of databases and knowledge resources available to individuals, organizations, schools of nursing, and health science libraries by modem through the Internet or via dial-in access. Subscribers to the Electronic Library have access to the following nursing knowledge resources:

- *Directory of Nurse Researchers* including biographical data about registered nurse researchers, a special database of researchers and projects funded by Sigma Theta Tau International; data gathered through the Survey of Nurse Researchers about registered research projects; and study descriptions and taxonomy descriptors;
- Research Conference Abstracts;
- Sigma Theta Tau International Grant Recipients and Projects;
- Information Resources Database;
- Table of Contents Database; and
- Gopher Searching Utility.

If you have access to a computer and a modem, you can "visit" the Electronic Library through its Internet address: telnet stit-sun.iupui.edu or you can use the dial-in number, (317) 687–2271. The voice telephone number is (317) 634–8171.

The American Nurses Association home page at http://www.nursingworld.org/index.htm guides readers to information about The American Nurses Association. Authorized ANA and state nurses association staff may access ANA * NET, the intranet for ANA and the state nurses association offices.

Disclaimer

As we complete this section on gathering information by using new technologies, we remind our readers to beware of useless or dangerous medical advice that appears online. Sam Uretsky, assistant director of pharmacy at New York University Medical Center and part-time consultant to the U.S. Postal Service Consumer Protection Service, addressed this issue in his article "Bad Medicine" appearing in *Internet World* in February 1996. His article states that some discussion groups are major sources of bad information. Because there is no cure for certain diseases, almost all sufferers look for something outside of conventional medicine to help relieve their pain:

> Posters on the Internet offer copper bracelets, magnets, honey, and diets that avoid tomatoes and peppers as treatment (for arthritis). None of these help, but they're posted with a great deal of assurance . . . As more people see the Internet as a way to spread commercial messages, there is an increasing number of quack ads in newsgroups . . . Before you trust your health to a Usenet posting, check up on it, double check, then check it again. (Uretsky, 1996, pp. 54–55)

Table 5.6. Selected Forums on CompuServe of Interest to Nurses

Forum	CompuServe (GO)
Attention Deficit Disorder: Information for parents of children with ADD, adults with ADD, those who work with or are married to someone with ADD, or those who are involved with a person with ADD in a professional context, such as physicians or therapists. A section discusses neurobehavioral disorders, such as Tourette's Syndrome.	GO ADD
Cancer Forum: Information about cancer. Support for those who have cancer and for their friends and relatives. No medical opinions.	GO CANCER
Diabetes and Hypoglycemia Forum: Information for those interested in diabetes, hypoglycemia and related chronic metabolic disorders.	GO DIABETES
Disabilities Forum: Information on developmental, mental, learning, deaf/hard of hearing, mobility and other disabilities.	GO DISABILITIES
Health & Fitness: Information on a wide range of interests involving health and fitness.	GO GOODHEALTH
Natural Medicine Forum: Information about natural medicine.	GO HOLISTIC
Medical: Information to help with use of computers in medicine. Contains a library section on nursing.	GO MEDSIG
Recovery: Information about varied areas of recovery including adult children, alcohol and drug recovery, nicotine, compulsive debt, and AIDS recovery.	GO RECOVERY
Safetynet: Information on any aspect of safety including occupational health, engineering, fire prevention, and law enforcement.	GO SAFETYNET

INTERVIEW EXPERTS

The latest information in your field may not be published in books, magazines, or journals. It might not even be available in computer databases or microfilm collections. Therefore, to write about current developments, unpublished information, or controversial matters, you will need to consult individuals who have special skills or knowledge derived from education, experience, or training—experts. These experts may be your colleagues. If so, consider interviewing them about their expertise on your topics.

> All writers must become good interviewers. There is no choice in the matter. Here's why. Non-fiction writers cannot write contemporary biographies unless they know how to thoroughly interview the people they wish to profile, as well as source people close to the ones being profiled. Furthermore, feature articles must be 'quote rich' in order to hold a reader's interest, and that means quotes must be obtained through interviews. Even facts for straight works of journalism are often gathered by interviewing researchers, eyewitnesses, civic leaders, or corporate executives. (Hensley, 1985, p. 12).

Direct questioning is helpful when you need facts about events and conditions with which the expert is knowledgeable or when you need statements about future actions, attitudes, opinions, or work in progress. Through interviewing, you can minimize misunderstandings because you can clarify each point with the experts. You can also pursue topics in depth and observe the experts' interaction with the topic. Interviewing experts allows you to go into greater depth about a topic than using questionnaires or surveys. Through interviews, you can probe for more complete data than otherwise. Moreover, by establishing rapport with the experts, you may set the stage for obtaining further insights.

Finding Experts

If there are no experts on your topic in your work setting, then begin seeking experts in your professional organization. Since most experts belong to professional associations, check the *Encyclopedia of Associations* for association names and addresses. The national organization may be able to help you find the expert for whom you are looking.

Locate nurses through ANA or NLN board members or specialty professional associations. The National League for Nursing provides advisory, analytical, interpretive, and referral information on nursing education, nursing practice, nursing staffing, and nursing-related health care issues.

If you know the name of an expert on your topic, use directories commonly found in libraries such as *Who's Who, Who's Who in American Nursing,* or *American Men and Women of Science.* You may be able to locate a university professor through the school's faculty directory or through the *National Faculty Directory.* Locate physicians through the *American Medical Directory* published by the American Medical Association.

If you do not have the specific name of an expert, then look in *Books in Print* and *Subject Guide to Books in Print.* The 1994–1995 edition of *Subject Guide to Books in Print* provides access by subject to all the nonfiction titles covered in *Books in Print.* It classifies more than 876,000 nonfiction titles under more than 74,000 Library of Congress subject headings. In addition, consult *Forthcoming Books in Print,* which lists over 170,000 soon-to-be published books with annotations annually. These will direct you to authors of books on your topic. You can contact book authors through their publishers or contact magazine authors through the magazines for which they write.

The *Research Centers Directory* lists university-related and other non-profit organizations that are conducting research. You can also consult faculty members at colleges and universities, the National Referral Center of the Library of Congress, museums, research institutes, government information centers, and laboratories.

If you need statistical information, you may want to contact government offices, corporations, colleges, banks, national unions, transportation companies, media, and other business services. Use *The National Directory of Addresses and Telephone Numbers* published in paperback by W. C. C. Directories. You can also consult out-of-town telephone directories found in most large public libraries or telephone company offices.

Getting Experts to Help You

After you locate experts, call them and let them know why you are contacting them. Be sure you have already completed a basic literature search and have exhausted other available resources. Let the experts know you would like to give them credit in your article and that they can review the article prior to its going to press. Ask them to send you any background material or article reports about themselves so that you can be better prepared for the interview. Know what you want so that you do not waste the experts' time.

Using Interviews

An interview is a method for collecting information in which you question respondents either face-to-face or by telephone. Successful interviews can be dynamic interpersonal experiences that give you the information for your manuscript and about complex topics that do not lend themselves to other types of information-gathering. Although there are various kinds of interviews, this chapter deals with unstructured interviews in which you have complete freedom to develop the interview in the most appropriate manner for the situation. In this type of interview, you use questions based on your knowledge and understanding of the issues you are addressing and encourage the experts to express their feelings and state their information.

When you arrange for an interview, do it well in advance of the time you will need the information to meet a deadline. Let the interviewee know about the agenda you are planning for the interview and ask for permission to tape the interview. Then send a confirmation letter about the arrangements and call to confirm a few days in advance.

Preparing for Interviewing

Before you interview the experts, find out as much as possible about the topic as well as about the people you will interview. Check the spelling of their names as well as their current position, title, and professional affiliation. To find out whether there is any previously published biographical material on the interviewee, check the *Biography and Genealogy Master Index*, published by Gale Research Company. This volume lists anyone included in any biographical index. Marquis' *Who's Who* is the best known biographical index and is actually a series of biographical indices. All *Who's Who* listings are in the *Master Index*.

As you prepare for the interviews, decide the scope of the topic you want to cover. Prepare questions with which you can draw out the experts about their experiences and specialized knowledge. Be sure to prepare questions prior to the interview. Use Figure 5.3 as your interview guide— write questions on it prior to the interview and complete as much as possible of the information prior to the interview. Check all information with the interviewee during the interview.

Analyze the topic sufficiently to plan a list of questions. Then review your questions to see if they deal with the complexities of your topic, if you have phrased them clearly and simply, and if they are biased.

Next, plan which questions you want to use first. The more questions you prepare, the more thorough your article will be. Save controversial questions for later in the session. Design open-ended questions rather than

Interviewee Contact Information

Name _____	Date _____
Title _____
Company/Affiliation _____
Address _____
Telephone(s) _____ Fax_____E-mail _____
Academic Background _____
Awards/Honors _____
Professional Organization Affiliations _____

The Interview

Date and Time of Interview _____
Address and Meeting Place _____
Directions to Interview Location _____

The Logistics

❑ Tape Recorder	❑ Extra Tape	❑ Batteries	❑ Extension Cord
❑ Note Pad	❑ Pencils and Pens	❑ Camera	❑ Extra Film
❑ Your business card	❑ Other		

The Article

The Article's Topic and Working Title
_____
_____
_____

The Questions

Create open-ended questions beginning with "Who, What, When, Why, Where, and How"
1. _____
2. _____
3. _____

Figure 5.3. Interview form (© 1995, Dowdney & Sheridan).

ones that can be answered easily by "yes" or "no," and ask "why" and "how" as much as the "who, what, when, and where." Unstructured, open-ended questions allow flexibility so that as interviewees say something that sounds interesting, you can explore the topic further. "What facet of cost-containment is most in need of investigation?" is an example of an open-ended question.

Create broad, general questions as well as narrow, specific ones. Keep your questions short and ask only one question at a time. Try to make your questions free of value judgments so that you present an impartial, unbiased approach. Try not to show surprise, disagreement, or agreement with what the individual says. Encourage candor by neither approving or disapproving.

Bring your watch, pens or pencils, a large notepad, and your business card so that the experts may contact you about new developments or new information on the topic. You also may want to bring a portable cassette tape recorder that works with batteries or electricity. Bring extra batteries, an extension cord, and an extra tape in case one tape is defective or one interview leads to a longer interview than you originally anticipated. If you plan to use a tape recorder, ask the interviewee's permission before you begin using it. You can do this while running the tape to have a record of the permission. Start with "Today's date is. . . . I, (your name), am interviewing (name of interviewee)." Ask the person to state that you have permission to tape this interview and use it for quotation in your article. Be sure to allow a full minute for the blank leader tape before you being the interview. Using a tape recorder during an interview has several benefits: you will have an accurate and complete record of everything said, including anecdotes; you can concentrate on the interview rather than on the note-taking process; and you can get more information in a shorter time.

Using a tape recorder has the disadvantage of potential mechanical problems. In addition, some interviewees may become self-conscious about being taped, thus inhibiting a free-flowing interview. Once you start the tape recorder, do not look at it. Instead, maintain eye contact with the person you are interviewing.

If you have some photographic expertise, bring a camera with black-and-white film to take pictures to illustrate your article. Often experts can supply you with a black-and-white glossy photograph. Be sure to find out whether or not they would like it returned.

Conducting Interviews

Arrive early for the interview so that you can observe your subject's surroundings and environment for added details. As you conduct the interview, use your sense of sight, hearing, taste, and touch because your senses will help you set the scene for your readers.

Use your sense of smell and taste to include details such as the aroma of coffee or tea, pipe smoke, or laboratory smells. Remember how the interviewee approaches you and shakes hands. Does the person seem distant and formal? Or friendly and casual? Identify yourself and the reason for the interview. Let the expert know what you hope to accomplish and why you selected him or her for the interview. Let the expert know how you will use the information and if a draft of the material will be available for review before publication. Also inform them about any deadline involved for providing follow-up information.

As you begin the interviews, establish rapport with the experts by helping them feel comfortable talking with you and sharing ideas. Review your purpose, and build an atmosphere of trust and respect. If you can help them feel relaxed, they will share their ideas with you more freely rather than answering your questions mechanically. Try to see things from their viewpoint. Remember, your purpose is not to debate, compete with, or share your own opinions with them.

To establish rapport, be pleasant, efficient, and poised, and use a straightforward manner. Beware of appearing either intimidated or patronizing to the expert. Don't fire questions as in a third-degree inquisition. Pace the questions according to the speed of response from the expert. Begin with general questions, followed by more specific ones. As you interview, be aware of your own tone of voice and expression so that you are not inadvertently influencing the expert's responses.

Listening intelligently to what they are saying is vital to good interviewing. As you listen, watch for their nonverbal communication. Observe gestures, and learn to read and decode silence as well as audible cues. Watch for how something is said by listening for inflections. Listen for hesitancy or enthusiasm in their manner of speaking. Watch how they sit in the chair, frown or smile, and move their head, hands, and feet. Maintain eye contact, concentrate on the expert, and accept any emotional content along with the verbal message. Observe their surroundings, and listen for memorable statements and direct quotes that will add flavor to your manuscript.

Barriers That Prevent Effective Interviews

Defensiveness and dogmatism on your part will hinder the interview's effectiveness. Avoid relating the information only to your own needs and viewpoints. Instead, concentrate on what the expert is saying so that you can listen from that frame of reference and from the reader's viewpoint.

Interrupting the interviewee can cut off communication. Lack of flexibility on your part can also hinder the interview. As you interview experts, give them freedom to express themselves in their own ways rather than using leading questions in which you suggest desirable or preferred answers. At the same time, follow the agreed-upon agenda so that time is not wasted.

Concluding Interviews

As you conclude your interview, ask about sources of additional information and other people to interview if applicable to your article. Contacting these other individuals will help you to balance the opinions and observations of your article's subject. If appropriate, prepare a transcript of the interview and request a written acknowledgment of its accuracy and permission to use it in your manuscript.

Telephone Interviews

You may also conduct interviews over the telephone. To do this, however, make prior arrangements with the individuals to be interviewed so that they will be expecting your call and prepared to give you the information you seek. Often, mailing a copy of the interview questions ahead is useful. Electronic devices are available for recording telephone conversations, but before using such devices, obtain permission from the interviewee for recording the conversation.

Although interviewing over the telephone is less costly than conducting in-person interviews, it may be a less effective information-gathering method because telephone interviews deny you the ability to build rapport in the same way you can in face-to-face interviews.

Question-and-Answer Framework for Articles

You may decide to develop your interview into a question-and-answer framework. Question-and-answer articles give your readers precise answers to basic questions about complex issues. This framework is ideal to use for controversial topics and personalities because your readers will hear ideas and quotations directly from the subject.

However, the interview format is not frequently used in the nursing literature and offers many opportunities to nurse authors. Think of some nurse leaders you know. What would you like to ask them? Wouldn't other nurses also like to know these answers? What journals do these other nurses read? The answer to these three questions may lead you to a wealth of topics and target markets.

Whether constructing an interview article or asking a few questions of a work colleague who is an expert on your topic, always confirm your quotations with your interviewee. This is especially true if the quotation was taken out of the context. Also, spend considerable time constructing clear, open-ended questions.

Networking

> Networking. . . . The cliché for cooperation . . . represents the purposeful seeking out of new and extensive relationships. It involves developing formal and informal support, advice giving, and informational systems among large numbers of groups and individuals . . . Networking establishes a rapid communication line, albeit informal and unofficial. One's networks play major parts in one's self-education system. (Stevens, 1985, p. 213)

"Informal information networks—grapevines, if you will—can be surprising, useful, and productive for a writer," said Kay Maria Porterfield (1984, p. 36). Her article, "Harvesting Fruit from the Writer's Grapevine," indicates several benefits of using networking: it gives you ideas; it makes your writing unique and fresh; it keeps you up to date on the writing profession; and it enables you to work smarter, not harder.

To make networking efficient, create a business card file of individuals who might be sources of specialized information. File the cards by the date you receive them and add background facts about the person who gave you the card.

Now that you have gathered a wealth of information from a wide variety of sources, you are ready to write your article. First, however, you need to organize the content, or your manuscript will face a high probability of extensive revisions—maybe nonsalvaging revisions. The next chapter, "Organize the Content," addresses the least talked about but biggest problem in writing.

EXERCISES

1. Gather information about your topic and complete your search.
2. Plan and schedule any necessary interviews.

REFERENCES

American library directory. (1994–1995). New York: R. R. Bowker Co.
American medical directory. (Annual) Chicago, IL: American Medical Association.
American men and women of science. (1995–1996). New York: R. R. Bowker.
Binger, J. (1981). The nursing journal–learning resource, professional symbol, and commodity. *Image, 13*(13), 67–70.
Biography and genealogy master index. (1995). Detroit, MI: Gale Research.
Books in print. (Annual). New York: R. R. Bowker Co.
Butler, M. (1994). *How to use the Internet.* Emeryville, CA: Ziff-Davis.
Cumulative index to nursing and allied health literature. (Annual). Glendale, CA: Cumulative Index to Nursing and Allied Health Literature Corp.
Eddings, J. (1994). *How the Internet works.* (pp. 9, 43–44). Emeryville, CA: Ziff-Davis.
Encyclopedia of associations. (Annual). Detroit, MI: Gale Research.
Fondiller, S. (1994, August). Writing for publication. *American Journal of Nursing, 94*(8), 62–64.
Forthcoming books in print. (Annual). New York: R. R. Bowker Co.
Grant, W. H. (1995). *Tech Notes.* The World Wide Web: The Internet unleashed.
Hahn, H. ,& Stout, R. (1995). *The Internet yellow pages.* Berkeley, CA: Osborne McGraw-Hill.
Hart, A. (1996, February). Second opinion. *Internet World,* 42.
Hensley, D. E. (1985). How to write interviews. *The Christian Writer, 4*(3), 12.
Hospital literature index. (Quarterly with annual cumulations). Chicago, IL: American Hospital Association.
Index medicus. (Monthly and annual cumulated index). Washington, DC: U.S. Government Printing Office.
International nursing index. (Quarterly with annual cumulations). New York: American Journal of Nursing Company.
James-Catalano, C. (1995, October). The good fight. *Internet World,* 34.
MaranGraphics. (1996). *Netscape 2 Simplified.* Foster City, CA: IDG Books.
Maraccio, K. Y., (Ed.). (1991). *Computer-readable databases: A directory and data sourcebook.* Detroit, MI: Gale Research.
National directory of addresses and telephone numbers. New York: W. C. C. Directories, Inc.
National faculty directory. (1995). Detroit, MI: Gale Research.
Nicholl, L. H. (1993, September). Managing bibliographic information. *Journal of Nursing Administration, 23*(9), 13–14.
Nichols, K. C. (1994). Bibliographic resources for medical communicators. In P. Minick (Ed.), *Biomedical communication: Selected AMWA workshops.* Bethesda, MD: American Medical Writers Association.
Nilson, J. N. (1995). *Bibliographic resources for medical communicators.* American Medical Writers Association Workshop, Asilomar, 37.
O'Keefe, S. (1995, October). Electric texts. *Internet World,* 58.
Porterfield, K. M. (1984, June). Harvesting fruit from the writer's grapevine. *Writer's Digest,* 36–38.
Research center directory. (1994). Detroit, MI: Gale Research Co.

Sheridan, D. R., & Dowdney, D. L. (1984). *Survey of selected nurse authors.* Unpublished work.

Squires, S. (1996, Winter). Experts talk about computer-assisted reporting. *Merck Media minutes.* 3.

Stevens, B. J. (1985). *The nurse as executive.* Rockville, MD: Aspen.

Subject guide to books in print. (Annual). New York: R. R. Bowker Co.

Uretsky, S. (1996, February). Bad medicine. *Internet World,* 54–55.

Westra, B. L., & Larsen, K. (1994, November). Saving time using C.I.N.A.H.L. on C.D.-R.O.M. *Nursing 94,* p. 94.

Who's who. (Annual). Chicago, IL: Marquis Who's Who, Inc.

Who's who in American nursing. (Annual). Chicago, IL: Marquis Who's Who, Inc.

6

Organize the Content

Now that you have developed a writing plan and gathered information through performing a literature search or interviewing an expert, you are probably eager to begin writing. That's great. But first you need to spend some time thinking—focusing your theme and organizing the content. Your goals in organizing your manuscript include identifying all relevant information and deciding on your priorities in presenting the information.

The most efficient step for you to take at this point is to focus your topic, then organize the facts you have gathered. It is much easier to write when you have identified key points. Good organization saves you time and work that otherwise will be needed later in revising your manuscript's structure. Besides, revising an unfocused, poorly organized manuscript can be difficult; sometimes such manuscripts are unsalvageable. One nurse author who claimed to be very unorganized said she does not outline, and that her manuscripts have a tendency to need a lot of editing and revisions. She also said that sometimes the thoughts never flow sequentially.

In her chapter "Formal Outlining for Writers and Editors" in *Biomedical Communication: Selected AMWA Workshops,* Elizabeth Whalen said:

> Justifiably or not, writing that has good potential is sometimes judged to be "bad" because the author lacks the ability to organize ideas. In scientific writing, especially, the illogical arrangement of ideas sometimes reflects negatively on the quality of thought. If the researcher has failed to write logically, how can the reader be sure that logical thinking guided the research? (Whalen, 1994, p. 34)

You will save yourself time and produce a better manuscript if you invest your time now in organizing the content into an outline. A manuscript will practically write itself from a well-organized outline. Outlines help you systematically arrange the topic so that a logical thread runs through the article. "Your first draft may be sketchy, but it will serve as a guideline to your note-taking. Without an outline you are likely to take notes on materials irrelevant to your purpose or overlook an idea which should be explored" (Van Alstyne, & Maddison, 1994, p. 363).

How can you pursue the creative part of the writing process and then move into the needed logical ordering of your information? The answer to this question is complex and not fully understood. Yet, knowing how to do this is essential to good writing.

When we asked selected nurse authors what process they used for writing, from idea to manuscript, most said thinking (creative) and outlining (logical) were important steps. Yet no respondent defined how to move from one to the other. That is probably because most of us are unclear about this part of our writing.

Moving through the creative to the logical phase of the writing process is often the greatest writing block for new writers, who wait for inspiration or believe they do not have the talent to write. Although talent or inspiration may work for some writers, we believe that each writer can move through these phases step by step with or without inspiration and talent.

Below are 10 steps we have developed that combine the best of many writing strategies. If you do not already have a strategy working for you, these 10 steps are a good way to move you through creativity to a detailed, orderly outline.

TEN-STEP PROCESS FOR ORGANIZING THE CONTENT

Through the following 10 steps you can focus your topic, integrate and organize the content (information you gathered), and select your target journal. These 10 steps will prepare you for fast, efficient writing. The 10 steps are:

1. Focusing the topic.
2. Listing the ideas.
3. Grouping the ideas.
4. Creating the diagrams.
5. Finding the framework.
6. Ordering the ideas.
7. Adding details.
8. Analyzing and revising the diagram.

9. Making a dash outline.
10. Creating a formal outline.

Step One: Focusing the Topic

Focus the working title by stating it as a sentence and then restating it as a question. The article you write will answer the question. You may have done this to derive your working title. If not, do it now. Focusing your topic is essential to the other nine steps. Be sure your topic is not too broad. Your working title determines what to include in the article.

For example, if someone selected the topic "Communication," this topic is large enough for a library of books rather than just one article. Begin narrowing the topic's focus to a more manageable size such as "Management Communication," then "Useful Management Communication with Quality Assurance Consultants." This latter specific topic could be developed into an article. Your goals in organizing your manuscript include identifying all relevant information and deciding on your priorities in presenting the information.

A second example of focusing a large topic into a manageable article is the subject of "Resumes." Several books have been written on this topic, but by narrowing it to "Resumes for Nurse Managers," the topic is now focused to be appropriate for publication. When focused even more clearly, Dowdney's final title for an article on this topic appeared in *Nursing Management* as "For Professional Advancement: Your Resume" (Dowdney, 1984).

Step Two: Listing the Ideas

Take a blank sheet of paper and write your focused topic at the top. Gather all the information you have collected from various sources. Then construct a long list of possible ideas you could include in your article. Your goal is to put ideas on paper; no order is necessary. Do not judge, just write ideas.

Several methods you could use in generating a list include brainstorming, asking and answering questions about your topic, dictating and transcribing random thoughts, pulling ideas from free-flow writing, and reviewing notes from library searching and interviews.

Brainstorming. You can generate many related ideas using brainstorming techniques. Many of the techniques suggested in Step Two are similar to those used in Chapter Two. In Chapter Two you generated ideas to find an article topic—here you are generating ideas about your topic.

Quickly jot down ideas related to your topic—as many as come into your head. Remember, in this type of free association, do not judge ideas; go for quantity, not quality; build new ideas off other ideas.

Asking and Answering Questions.   Add to your list by asking yourself questions about your topic. Begin questions with *who, what, when, where, why,* and *how?* For example, let's say that you plan to write about family education for patients with progressive dementia and that you plan to deal with nursing care, causes, and stages. Begin by asking questions such as "Who gets progressive dementia?" "Who takes care of these people?" You can add the answers as you develop your list, but you do not need to put them in their ultimate order. In fact, you do not even need to write complete sentences at this point. Just generate a long list of ideas answering the questions related to your topic. Do not stop to look up facts; instead, write clues so you can look up facts later, such as "find definition," "find statistics," or "write personal experience." Use key words that remind you of personal experiences such as anecdotes about patients. Ask more questions and continue to add ideas to your list.

Dictating and Transcribing Random Thoughts.   Barbara Brown, editor of *Nursing Administration Quarterly,* said in a 1980 presentation at Stanford University Hospital that speaking into a tape recorder's microphone is one of her favorite methods of drafting articles or editorials. You can use this method now to generate related ideas or in Chapter Eight when you write the manuscript. If you use this method now, dictate your ideas freely. Irene Heywood Jones (1983) wrote, "I invested in a cassette recorder to capture evasive and invaluable impromptu flashes" (p. 46). After dictating, have the information transcribed as a list with spaces between ideas.

Pulling Ideas from Free-Flow Writing.   Another method that is similar to dictating is writing random thoughts using the free flow method explained in Chapter One. This is a particularly good technique to use if you are trying to deal with writer's block. Just sit down and keep writing for 10 minutes about your topic. Write anything, but do not stop. If something else keeps popping into your head, write that too. Then return to your topic. After you finish, take a colored pen and circle the ideas related to your topic. Add them to your list.

Reviewing Notes from Library Searching and Interviews.   Your most obvious sources of ideas are the notes you took at the library, interview transcripts, or collateral materials you may have obtained such as a policy statement or committee minutes. Consult as many sources as possible to ensure that you present facts rather than opinions. If you are stating opinions, be accurate and state them as opinions, and identify the person whose opinions they are. Read all your materials to "stuff your brain." Then put them aside and add the ideas that seemed most relevant or important to your list. You can go back to your sources later for exact information where needed, but first put it through your brain once. This technique will help you internalize the material, sort out the parts you need, and help you to integrate rather than "lift" borrowed information. Of course, you need to give credit for information you borrowed from other sources. (See the topic of plagiarism in Chapter Eight.) Sift through your brain all the material related to your article, do not just copy.

Now that you have used some or all of the above techniques, you should have generated and written a substantial list of ideas about your topic. It is fine for now that there is no order to these thoughts. The next several steps address ordering. Put your list aside for a day, then bring it out and add more ideas. Continue to add to your list as you work through later steps of the Process.

Step Three: Grouping the Ideas

Spread out your pages of lists and add any highlighted article pages and note cards. Look at all your ideas to see whether some form natural groups. For instance, if you see you have written about various symptoms, products, results, or elements of historical background, think about whether these could form a logical grouping. If some categories or natural groupings occur, mark similar items with colored pens. (For example, place a red dot before all the symptoms, products, results, or historical background on your lists.) Do not force items into a group; just look for those that occur naturally.

Step Four: Creating the Diagrams

Using diagrams as organizing concepts is gaining popularity in teaching thinking, writing, and organizing skills because it allows for a creative process in a somewhat structured way. Diagrams have been called "spoke outlines," "clusters," "issue trees," "patterns," and "maps." We call our diagrams "Sun Diagrams."

Each of these diagramming strategies will help you synthesize your ideas, generate words easily, organize articles efficiently, and write coherently. After explaining the highlights of several diagramming methods, we will show you the details involved in creating Sun Diagrams.

Spoke Outline. In *Overcoming Writing Blocks* (1979), Mack and Skjei introduced the spoke outline. The theme is placed in the center and supporting ideas on spokes emanating from the center as the ideas emanate from the theme. This ordering scheme allows the writer to escape the problems of the more traditional outline model. It graphically reflects the incompleteness and absence of hierarchical order in your thinking at the early stages of the writing process, and it gives you room to easily expand, contract, or rearrange the elements of the outline. At the same time, it lends a preliminary form to your job.

As you work with diagrams, you begin seeing relationships and connections between ideas. Later the diagram becomes sequenced—what comes first, second, and so forth. When you have not thought through your ideas, you will begin seeing gaps in the logic. A good diagram will point out these gaps clearly so that you can address them.

Mindmaps. "A mindmap is a drawing in which you place all the main ideas of your information and draw connections between them. Mindmapping lets you work out the hierarchical relationships of the information without worrying about the order (Fawcett, Ferdinand, & Rockley, 1993, p. 60).

Hypertext and Information Mapping®. In *Mapping Hypertext*, Robert Horn stated:

> For a number of years I have been working with two relatively new frameworks for improving human communication. They are:
>
> **Hypertext**—A form of organizing text in computers that permits the linking of any place in text (or other media) to any other place and the rapid retrieval of information by following trails of these associative links.
>
> **Information Mapping's Method of Structured Writing**—a methodology for analyzing, organizing, writing, sequencing, and formatting information to improve communication. It provides a way of describing the structure of subject matters that is very useful throughout the communication process. (Horn, 1989, Introduction)

Clustering. Because the diagramming process pulls together related ideas, Rico called the process "clustering." Clustering is a nonlinear brainstorming process similar to free association. It uses a nonlinear association process that allows patterns to emerge. This diagram places a major theme in the center and develops it by connecting it to random thoughts.

> Through clustering we naturally come up with a multitude of choices from a part of our mind where the experiences of a lifetime mill and mingle. It is the writing tool that accepts wondering, not-knowing, seeming chaos, gradually

mapping an interior landscape as ideas begin to emerge. It is an openness to the unknown . . . it acknowledges that it's okay to start writing not knowing exactly what, where, who, when, and how. Most writers acknowledge that this is how it inevitably is anyway (Rico, 1983, pp. 28–29).

Issue Trees. Linda Flower (1985) described the writing process by using an "issue tree," which is a sketch that resembles an upsidedown tree and that places ideas in a hierarchical order.

Issue trees have two main things to offer writers. First, they let you sketch or test out ideas and relationships as you write. At the same time they let you visualize the whole argument and see how all the parts might fit together. Issue trees can also help you generate new ideas. A traditional outline, written before you start the paper, only arranges the facts and ideas you already know. An issue tree highlights missing links in your argument and helps you draw inferences and create new concepts (Flower, 1985, pp. 95–96).

Patterning. Tony and Robbie Fanning use "patterning," similar to the spoke diagram, in their book, *Get It All Done and Still Be Human* (1979). They suggest that "patterning mirrors the way your brain creates ideas. The whole point of patterning is to capture information and ideas as they're generating without trying to organize them first. . . . It is an effective, fast way to gather and externalize your thoughts" (Fanning & Fanning, 1979, p. 7).

The Sun Diagram. The Sun Diagram is a creative visual writing tool that look like a sun radiating light beams. In the center of the sun you will write your article's theme; then you will write ideas radiating from the theme on the rays.

To create a Sun Diagram, take a large sheet of paper from a flipchart pad or use continuous computer paper. Write your focused theme in the center. Then draw lines from the center so that they look like the rays from the sun. These are your primary rays. On these rays, write your main ideas beginning with those ideas that you have grouped together. Related items go together on rays with their group label (whatever these ideas are called collectively). Supporting ideas are branched off major rays (see Figure 6.1).

Look for possible patterns or relationships; there are no right or wrong ways to create the diagrams. Using a diagram is a right-brain, creative activity similar to designing.

Rico described the process:

The thought pattern characteristic of the right brain lends itself to the formation of original ideas, insights, discoveries. We might describe it as the kind

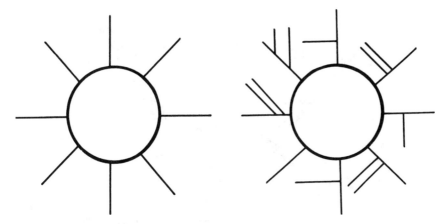

Figure 6.1. Basic sun diagrams (© 1983 Dowdney & Sheridan).

of thought prevalent in early childhood, when everything is new and everything has meaning. . . . Your Design mind has perceived connects and has made a pattern of meaning. It takes the logical, rational acts and facts of the world you know, the snippets of your experience, the bits and pieces of your language capabilities, and perceives connections, patterns, and relationships in them. While the right brain does this naturally, it is often overpowered by the logical, critical processes of the left brain. (Rico, 1983, pp. 261–262)

Beware of your critical left brain and allow yourself some space for creativity as you design a Sun Diagram for your manuscript. Remember, there is no right or wrong way to construct your diagram because you are taking a creative step.

Write your question in the center. Then put key ideas on rays from the center. The rays are places for examples, ancillary statements, and tangential concepts. Draw several Sun Diagrams, and organize each one differently.

One other technique that may allow you to try more ways to organize is to write your key ideas on tiny papers that have sticky adhesive backs that allow them to be easily removed. Move the ideas (papers) into different structures. If you use this technique, be sure to copy good arrangement possibilities before you rearrange them. The first Sun Diagram (Figure 6.2) was taken from an early stage of Donna Dowdney's article, "For Professional Advancement: Your Resume." The next Sun Diagram shows the ideas in a later stage—a more clustered arrangement. After clustering ideas, the ideas are put into sequential order with numbers.

Figure 6.3 shows early organization of content on "Assessing Current Management Development Needs" (Sheridan & Spector, 1985). That Sun

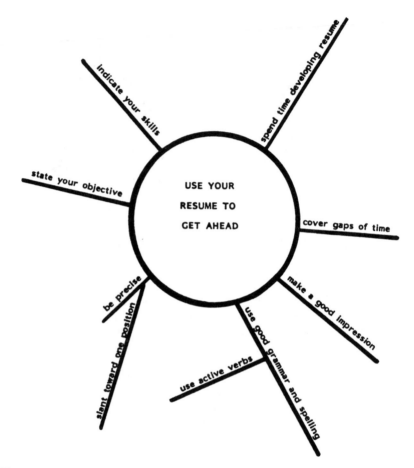

Figure 6.2. Arranging, clustering, and sequencing ideas (© 1985 Dowdney & Sheridan).

Diagram shows sidebars—the survey forms will accompany the article as separate sidebars.

Many other possible ways to organize this material would also have been appropriate. Do not look for the "right" one, but continue trying new arrangements until you find a clear organization. You may want to draw a few and then leave them for a day. Then draft a few more without looking at your initial diagrams.

One way to learn how to create a Sun Diagram is to analyze a few published articles by creating Sun Diagrams for them. After you read an article, state the article's topic, purpose, and title. Use this to find the article's theme. Put the theme or title (if it is representative of the theme) in the center. Then

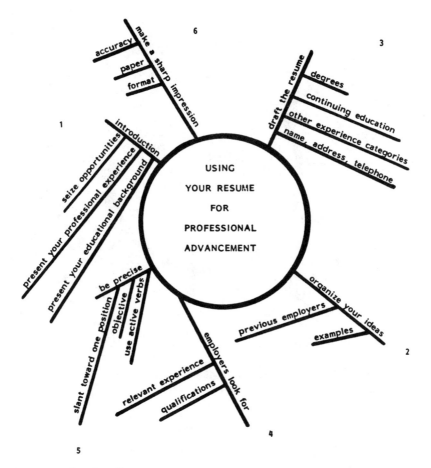

Figure 6.2. *(continued).*

look at the article's headings. Put the article's key points on rays emanating from the sun. Arrange the subtopics on subrays on lines off the key points' rays. Add new rays and draw new lines branching from each ray. These indicate places for examples, ancillary statements, and tangential concepts.

Step Five: Finding the Framework

All articles need frameworks. Figure 6.4 shows analysis of the framework of an article. Which type of framework to use is determined by the target journal requirements and your article's content. The first variable to consider is your target journal's requirements.

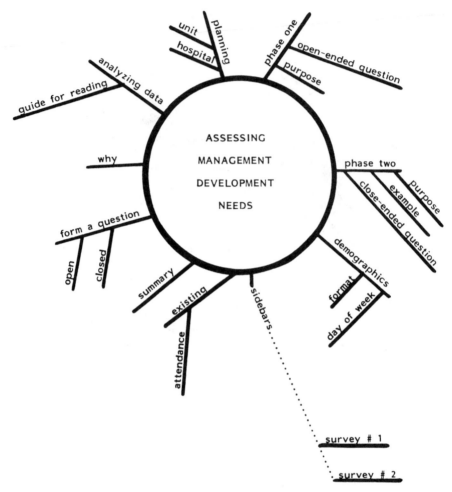

Figure 6.3. Sun diagram with sidebars (© 1983 Dowdney & Sheridan).

For instance, if you are writing for *RN*, you may use a natural evolved framework. That framework is not appropriate, however, for *Nursing Research*. Conversely, a research format sent to *RN* would also preclude your chances of being published because *RN* is a general nursing, easy reading magazine, and your submitted article must comply. As you select an organizing framework, consider both clarity and functionality, and be sure it matches your target journal's preferred format.

Examine the journal to which you plan to submit your manuscript so that you can determine the kinds of frameworks that journal prefers.

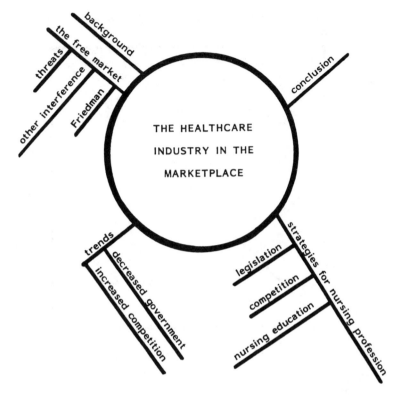

Figure 6.4. Analysis of an article's framework (© 1983 Dowdney & Sheridan).

Notice how the articles are organized and the kinds of headings and sidebars the journal uses. Creating a Sun Diagram on an article from your target journal could help you understand the frameworks used. Look at several other articles in that journal. Are they similar?

We have designed Figure 6.5 to show a continuum of writing frameworks. The four types of frameworks the continuum explains includes:

- The imposed specific framework (Figure 6.5A)
- The selected general framework (Figure 6.5B)
- The selected specific framework (Figure 6.5C)
- The evolved natural framework (Figure 6.5D)

Imposed Specific Framework. Some journals impose a specific framework. For example, if you are reporting on research, usually certain headings must be followed. These headings reflect the framework used.

Figure 6.5. Continuum of writing frameworks with examples (© 1985 Dowdney & Sheridan).

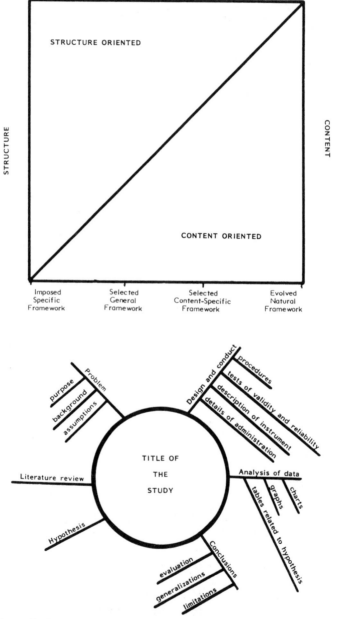

A. Imposed specific framework (Example: Research framework).

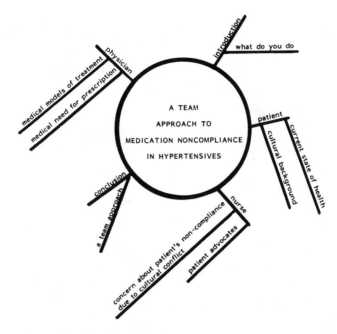

B. Selected general writing framework.

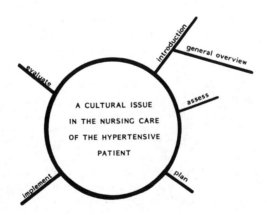

C. Selected content-specific framework.

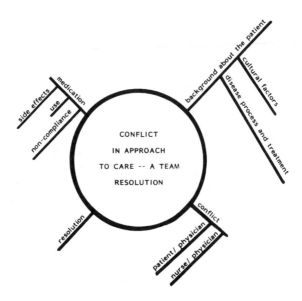

D. Evolved natural framework.

If you are writing for *Nursing Research,* use a research framework. Creativity in a framework is undesirable because it will lead to either rejection or extensive rewriting later. *Nursing Research* wants a research format. The research report generally includes six sections: formulation of the problem; review of the literature; hypothesis; design and conduct of the study; analysis of the data; and conclusions. Even though you may change the number of sections in a research manuscript, the content remains the same (see Figure 6.5A, Research Framework).

Treece and Treece (1973) describe the sections. Formulation of the problem includes purpose, background, and assumptions:

> Often a broad approach to the review of the literature is preferable to a narrow viewpoint that cites a few studies in detail. . . . The hypothesis should be explicit. It may be stated in either the null form or the working form. The null form does not suggest the end result, whereas the working hypothesis predicts the anticipated result. (p. 257)

The section on design contains "all details related to procedure. It describes the instrument, gives details of administration, considers tests of validity and reliability, and gives information concerning the sample" (Treece & Treece, 1973, p. 257).

In the section on analysis of the data, "tables developed for those items judged relevant to the hypothesis are necessary Discussion of the tables should precede their placement on a page. Tables, graphs, and charts are preferable to prose descriptions" (Treece & Treece, 1973, p. 258).

The conclusion

provides a synthesis of the findings and relates the various aspects of the study to the discipline in general. The conclusion of the report is not a place for new material, but a place for comprehensive evaluation and generalizations. The limitations of the study are included in the final chapter. . . . Other topics of the final chapter are implications and recommendations for further study. (Treece & Treece, 1973, p. 258)

Each of these six sections represents one ray radiating from your Sun Diagram. The framework for reports in a research journal may sometimes combine some of these sections or add a section such as a theoretical framework. Look at several articles in your target journal to determine the framework for research articles.

Your purpose in writing a research article is "not to demonstrate research competence but rather to communicate the contribution that the study makes to knowledge. Because readers are particularly interested in the findings of a research project, a relatively large proportion of the journal report is devoted to the results and discussion sections" (Polit & Hungler, 1983, p. 576).

Some nursing journals that publish research include *Nursing Research, Advances in Nursing Science, Research in Nursing and Health,* and the *Western Journal of Nursing Research.*

Preparing the written report is the final and most important step in the research process. . . . The report should present sufficient detail about the design and methodology to allow another investigator to replicate the study. (Southby, 1981, p. 719)

Technical and scientific journals that do not directly emphasize nursing also publish articles from nurses. Such journals may also have rigid mandatory frameworks to follow. If you send an article built around a creative content-oriented framework to a journal with a preferred format, you are almost assured a letter of rejection.

Two less extreme frameworks exist between the evolved natural framework and the imposed specific framework. If the journal does not specify a format, these are two ways you can organize your ideas by selecting a framework rather than evolving one the natural way. These formats offer ways to help you sort out your ideas onto your diagram.

Selected General Framework. A selected general framework is a structure you select that could be used for almost any topic. For example, ask questions—*who, what, when, where, why,* and *how.* Put one question on each ray of a Sun Diagram and sort out and organize your ideas onto the subrays according to which question they answer. Reporters use this framework in writing news stories. Other examples of general writing frameworks are shown in Figure 6.6.

Dichotomous frameworks (Figure 6.6) offering only two major rays include pro/con and before/after. These also need "introduction" and "summary," "conclusion," or "follow-up" rays. You simply fill in your content. Figure 6.7 shows an example of an article written on a dichotomous framework.

You can also use the problem-solving method in which you put one step on each ray. For example, define a problem, criteria for solution, alternatives, selection of solution, implementation of solution, and evaluation of solution. Or more simply, state the problem, write and expand on the solution and include supporting information in sidebars (Figure 6.7).

Perspectives could be used as a framework by putting a person or group on each ray—for example, nurse, patient, physician, family, etc. An introduction and conclusion could also be included, as well as some other rays such as background or issue.

Other popular frameworks in contemporary journals are the "steps" or "perspectives" frameworks, which are especially useful for "how-to" articles. For example, to learn how to break down barriers to creativity and begin with an open mind, McMillan (1985) wrote "10 Steps to Creativity" in *Nursing Success Today.* Similarly, historical or development articles use a sequential framework such as what happened first, second, third, etc. For example, in *"The American Journal of Nursing* and the Socialization of a Profession 1900–1920," Wheeler (1985) began with "purpose and method" and "significance." Then she organized the content by decades. Those subtitles were: "First Decade: 1900–1910" and "Second Decade: 1910–1920" (Wheeler, 1985). Another example, in "How to Plan and Carry Out Your Poster Session," was organized into the subheadings of "Week One, Week Two. . . . Week Eight." Supplementary information was provided on sidebars about "Advertising Principles, Glossary of Production Terms and Tips" (Morra, 1984).

An example of a "perspectives framework" appears in Figure 6.6. Case studies may also use this approach. For example, in the article "Help! She's Been Shot" (Clutter, Easter, Gloe, & Kiner, 1994) the story is relayed from the author's perspective: "In his eight years as a field paramedic, Steve thought he had encountered every conceivable medical emergency . . .". The story tells of the care of a patient with a facial gunshot from the perspective of four nurses.

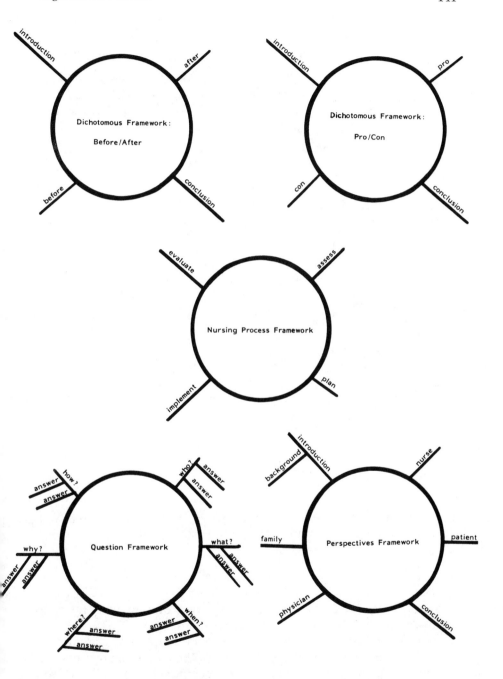

Figure 6.6. Framework examples (Dowdney & Sheridan © 1983).

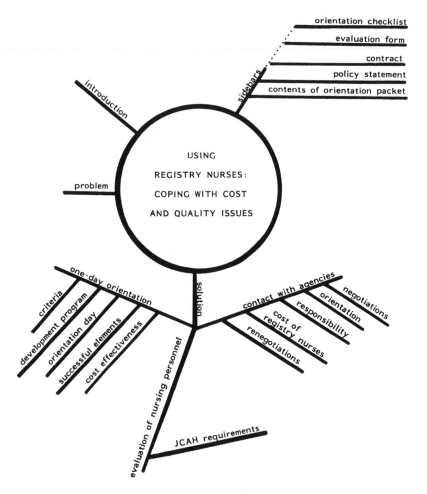

Figure 6.7. Dichotomous Framework: Problem/solution. Statement of problem with development of solution for article's content. (Sheridan & Dowdney © 1983).

Selected Specific Framework. Another type of framework for organizing your ideas is the selected specialty framework. This is a framework you select based on specific content. For example, if you are writing about marketing, you may use the steps of the marketing process. Remember, if you borrow someone's framework, be sure to give them credit with a citation.

One obvious framework to use is the nursing process (Yura & Walsh, 1978). Each step of the process (assess, plan, implement, evaluate) is put on a ray (Figure 6.6).

Sometimes a more medical model is used such as "pathophysiology, diagnosis, treatment, prognosis," etc. If you use a medical framework, be sure to add "nursing care" if you are writing for a nursing journal.

Another content-specific framework might be management functions such as planning, organizing, directing, and controlling. If you are writing about a management topic such as time management, you could use this framework to organize your material. For example, you might write about how to save time in performing each of your management responsibilities. Often you can select a framework to sort out your facts, organize your materials, and enrich your articles.

Suzanne Hall Johnson suggested in "Developing an Article Using the Nursing Model" that " most articles describing a project could be outlined within the sections of introduction, problem, goals, purpose, techniques, project evaluation" (Johnson, 1982, p. 58).

In writing nursing articles, you can organize your material by putting nursing action headings directly onto the rays of your Sun Diagram. Write an introduction emphasizing the nursing responsibility. Assess the patient (include what to assess for and pathophysiology), determine the need for therapy, provide safe nursing care, prevent complications, teach patient and family, evaluate, and summarize. In the summary, emphasize the importance of nursing care. Subheadings under "Provide Safe Nursing Care" may include nursing techniques, treatments, pictures, examples of patients and nursing care, showing "how to" pharmacology information, and care plans showing steps and rationale. Subheadings under "Prevent Complications" may be listed in a sidebar. Also, examples may fit here. Under the subheading "Teach Patient and Family," describe what to teach and techniques to use (Johnson, 1982).

An example of this organization is "Florence Nightingale: Yesterday, Today, and Tomorrow." The authors (Dennis & Prescott, 1985) organized the article using the obvious sequential framework—yesterday, today, and tomorrow. However, they also considered "Prevention and Promotion: Obscurity of the Sick," "Physical Environment," "Interpersonal and Psychological Milieu," and "Good Nursing: Its Facilitators and Directors." The article begins with "The Study," then considers "Yesterday," then each factor above is considered in light of yesterday and today. The last subheading is "Tomorrow." Figure 6.8 shows how this would look on a Sun Diagram.

Sometimes combining two frameworks is more easily planned on a grid before using the Sun Diagram. Plot one framework on each axis and fill in

	Yesterday	Today	Tomorrow
Prevention and Promotion	2	3	
Physical Environment	4	5	
Interpersonal and Psychological Milieu	6	7	
Good Nursing	8	9	
			10

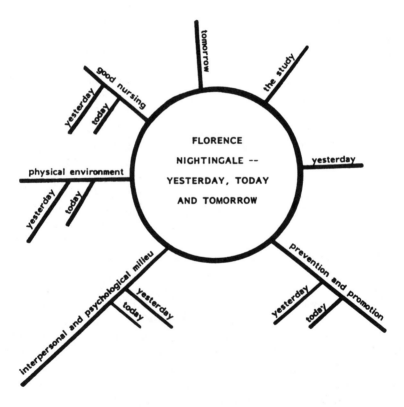

Figure 6.8. Two ways to organize the same information. *Top:* Grid framework. *Bottom:* Sequential framework (Dowdney & Sheridan © 1985).

information as needed. The above article planned on a grid is shown in Figure 6.8. "The Study," an essential introduction, is added prior to #1.

The numbers indicate the sequence of topics—they could be written in vertical order also, such as all yesterday, all today, all tomorrow. However, with little included about tomorrow, the organizational sequence is well selected for the content.

Be creative in looking for and developing frameworks. The same article may be written many ways in any number of frameworks. Unless you have an imposed format such as nursing research, you can develop your article using any of the frameworks on the continuum.

For example, you want to write about a patient you cared for who was noncompliant in taking his medication for hypertension. You discovered he would not take the medication because of the libido side effects. A discussion with him centered around elements of his Latin American "macho" cultural expectations, beliefs, and self-image. (There's more to the story, but that's enough for our purposes here.) How can this story be organized? You might cluster the ideas of the story in various ways to develop a series of diagrams. The organization of the content might evolve into a diagram such as the Evolved Natural Framework in Figure 6.5. Or you might organize it using a content-specific framework such as the nursing process. Your Sun Diagram might begin to look like the Selected Content-Specific Framework in Figure 6.5

You also could select a general writing framework such as perspectives. You would write the name of each person or group on a ray and sort your information into these categories. An introduction and conclusion will also be necessary. Your diagram might look something like the Selected General Writing Framework in Figure 6.5

Evolved Natural Framework. By allowing your right brain creativity to move the ideas around, you are developing a natural framework for your article. Like the framework of a house, your manuscript's framework needs to be clear and strong enough to give structural support. Sometimes frameworks evolve naturally from a manuscript's content. Natural frameworks evolve using the clustering of ideas followed by a series of Sun Diagrams as described above. Each article's natural framework is unique to the content of that article (see Sun Diagrams in Figure 6.5).

Step Six: Ordering the Ideas

After you have transferred your ideas onto rays and subrays, look for an order to the overall diagram. Which ray comes first, second, and so forth? Number the rays.

The order of the rays may be obvious, such as the steps of a procedure or the order of the nursing process. You may have a historical ordering—what happened first, second, third, etc. Other orders may include developmental, young to old, or progressive stages of a disease or phases of a project. Another article might show cause and effect. Some articles do not have as obvious an order; you will need to search for a logical sequence.

When you have determined the order of the rays, be sure they fit together. Draw a bridge from ray one to ray two. On this bridge, write words that tie the two rays together. Repeat, constructing a bridge between rays two and three, and so forth until you have connected all the rays. Any gaps in information in your article will become obvious as you try to connect the rays. Point number one may connect to two, but two may not connect to three without writing a lengthy transition on your bridge between two and three. This is an indication that you need to fill in this gap by creating a new ray. Then add a transitional bridge between the new ray and existing rays, reordering if necessary.

Step Seven: Adding Details to the Diagram

If you were writing a 500-word manuscript, each ray could represent a paragraph or a complete thought. If, however, you were writing a more lengthy manuscript, each ray might represent a section. To develop each section of the manuscript in more detail, copy what is written on one ray of your Sun Diagram into the center of a new sun. Make a new Sun Diagram for each ray of your primary diagram. Develop the ideas for each section on your diagrams. You should have one new Sun Diagram for each ray of your primary diagram. By using a secondary Sun Diagram, you allow for more complete development of your secondary sun outline's subparts. This process will help you develop the subparts in full. Again, gaps and odd rays will become apparent. On your secondary Sun Diagrams, each ray will represent a thought, usually a future paragraph or two. Now you have a detailed outline for your manuscript that reflects a theme (the center), an organizing framework (the rays), subtopics (on the rays), and transitions between subtopics (bridges).

Step Eight: Analyzing and Revising the Diagram

After you complete your diagram, put it away for several days. When you bring it out, make changes to refine it or try to draw it from memory and compare the two; this will help you rethink the organization of the diagram. Another method for reviewing your diagram is to tell a colleague about your manuscript as you draw and use your diagram as a guide while you are talking. Fill in the diagram, invite questions, and fill in any gaps based on your colleague's questions. Revise your diagram as necessary after others give you new insights.

Your Sun Diagram will help you diagnose and correct four common writing problems that are easy to correct at this point and difficult to correct later: 1) too broad a topic; 2) unrelated thoughts; 3) major gaps in logic or sequence; and 4) no connection between thoughts. These problems are visually obvious and easy to correct, whereas later in the writing process they are more difficult to identify and will take more work to correct.

You can tell if your topic is too broad if its rays do not have a natural end and if the diagram seems to go on endlessly. If this happens, you probably have several possible articles rather than only one.

To correct the problem of having too broad a topic, select one ray as your article. Put other rays back into your idea file for later articles. A less satisfactory way to correct this problem is to write an overview article that presents a broad range of subject matter without depth. However, most journals do not want this type of article.

If you have one or two unrelated thoughts, you will see this immediately when you try to order your rays and write transitions. You can deal with unrelated thoughts by looking at each ray in relation to the central theme in the sun. If any ray is unrelated, either delete or revise it. Learn to delete unrelated ideas or writing. If you feel reluctant to delete the idea, place the idea in your idea file for another article.

If the same word or idea appears on all of the rays, move that word to the center. It is part of your article's theme. After you have eliminated unrelated ideas, review your order and transitions. Look for a smooth logical sequence. There should be a thread of logic running through your diagram. This is the idea contained in the center of your Sun Diagram. Any idea unrelated to the sun does not belong in this article.

You may want to write your article directly from your Sun Diagram if you have developed subtopic Sun Diagrams. If, however, you prefer writing from a formal outline, or if the content in the Sun Diagram is still confusing to you, take the time to develop your diagram into an outline using the following two steps.

Step Nine: Making A Dash Outline

An outline has two interacting purposes. One is to shape the technical information in logical order. The other is to help organize your thinking. As you gradually construct an outline, it should oscillate between these two purposes until it settles down to an idealized compromise. Thus, the best way to work with an outline is to keep it flexible. The worst way is to consider it a rigid form into which you must fit your ideas and results (Michaelson, 1990, p. 140)

The dash outline uses dashes to indicate topics and orders the main rays, but does not order the subparts of the outline chronologically. List each ray as a Roman numeral in the order assigned. Write ideas from each ray under the ray heading. The framework for this is shown in Figure 6.9

Do not use complete sentences in a dash outline. After you include all your ideas, begin numbering the subpoints in this outline logically or chronologically. You can take this preliminary organization and use it to develop the formal outline.

Step Ten: Creating a Formal Outline

Like a road map, an outline indicates a starting point and keeps you moving logically so that you don't get lost before arriving at your conclusion. (Errors in logic are much easier to detect in an outline than in a draft). Using an outline makes larger and more difficult subjects easier to handle by breaking them into manageable parts; therefore, the less certain you are about your writing ability or about your subject, the fuller your outline should be. The parts of an outline are easily moved about, so you can experiment to see what arrangements of your ideas is the most effective. Perhaps most important, creating a good outline frees you to concentrate on writing when you begin the rough draft (by forcing you to organize your subject and structure your thinking beforehand). (Brusaw, Alred, & Oliu, 1993)

You are now ready to prepare a formal outline. There are two types of formal outlines. One uses Roman numerals. The other uses decimals, as shown in Figure 6.9 A,B,&C. Formal outlines have been taught for years as a writing tool—with good reason. Outlines lead readers by the shortest path to the information they need. Diagrams and outlines clearly point out flaws in order and gaps before you write. Parallelism, or its absence, becomes obvious.

Elizabeth Whalen reminds readers in her chapter on Formal Outlining for Writers and Editors to try to

use parallel language structure for all entries in our outline. This method focuses your thoughts on the logical progression of ideas rather than on writer's or editor's anxiety that causes blocks. If you are using a topic outline, decide which grammatical structure each entry requires (e.g., an infinitive phrase or a noun clause). In a word outline, the part of speech most often used for entries is a noun; however, whichever part of speech you choose (e.g., verb), use it consistently. Believe it or not, forcing yourself to retain the parallel structure enhances thinking about the topic and makes writing easier when

A: The Dash Outline
I. Introduction
   —xxxxxxxxxxxxxxxxxxxxxxxxxxxx
   —xxxxxxxxxxxxxxxxxxxxxxxxxxxx
II. Problem
III. Solution
IV. Method
   —xxxxxxxxxxxxxxxxxxxxxxxxxxxx
   —xxxxxxxxxx
V. Results
   —xxxxxxxxxxxxxxxxxxxxxxxxxxxxxx
   —xxxxxxxxxxxxxx
VI. Summary
   —xxxxxxxxxxxxxx
   —xxxxxxxxxxxxxxxxxxxxxxxxxxxxxxx

B: The Roman Numeral Outline
I. The first important idea (Use a key idea on one ray of the Sun Diagram)
   A. The first sub idea of ray 1.
      1. A point about A.
         a. First subpoint of 1.
            1) First subpoint of 1a.
            2) Second subpoint of 1a.
         b. Second subpoint of 1.
         c. Third subpoint of 1.
         d. Fourth subpoint of 1.
      2. Second point about A.
         a. First subpoint of 2.
            1) First subpoint of 2a.
            2) Second subpoint of 2a.
            3) Third subpoint of 2a.
         b. Second subpoint of 2.
      3. A third point about A.
   B. The second sub idea of I.
      1. First point about B.
      2. Second point about B.
II. The second important idea (Use a key idea on a second ray of the Sun Diagram)
   A. The first sub idea of ray II.
   B. The second sub idea of ray II.

C: The Decimal Outline
   1. The first important idea (Use a key idea on one ray of the Sun Diagram)
      1.1. The first sub idea of ray 1.
      1.2. The second sub idea of ray 1.
         1.2.1. The first subpoint of ray 1.2
         1.2.2. The second subpoint of ray 1.2
   2. The second important idea (Use a key idea on a second ray of the Sun Diagram)
      2.1. The first sub idea of ray 2.
      2.2. The second sub idea of ray 2.
   3. The third important idea (Use a key idea on a third ray of the Sun Diagram)
      3.1. The first sub idea of ray 3.
      3.2. The second sub idea of ray 3.

Figure 6.9. *A:* The Dash Outline; *B:* The Roman Numeral Outline; *C:* The Decimal Outline.

you draft the manuscript. A sentence outline, of course, imposes it own parallelism, and construction of a sentence outline facilitates the transition to writing your draft (Whalen, 1994, p. 35).

Furthermore, it is easy to write an article following a formal outline. Although it is difficult to develop an outline from scratch, it is not difficult to develop one from a Sun Diagram or a dash outline.

The cornerstone in developing an organized writing system is the outline. It is not essential that this tool be all-encompassing—in many cases this would be most unrealistic. However, an outline, however 'skeleton-like' guides and provides direction to the writer. The outline frequently goes through developmental stages as the writing process proceeds (Burkhalter, 1976, pp. 54–56)

Pamela Burkhalter described the stages as including major headings and subheadings. As the writer enlarges the outline, parts are deleted or condensed as the literature survey is continued. Thus, the outline becomes the writer's map during the writing phase.

The traditional Roman numeral outline (Figure 6.9B) follows a pattern of alternating letters and numbers to show subordination of ideas. The various parts of the outline also may be the same as the headings you use in your manuscript.

Using formal outlining gives you a starting point. It helps you organize your thoughts, reveals flaws, and shows gaps in logical sequences. Formal outlines use parallel grammatical structure, begin with Roman numeral I, and alternate with capital letters, numbers, and lowercase letters. You can develop your formal outline from your dash outline or from a detailed Sun Diagram. To go from a dash outline to a formal outline, order the main headings (each ray) with a Roman numeral; subheadings with capital letters; next lower level data with 1,2,3, and so forth. In summary, to construct a formal outline using Roman numerals directly from your Sun Diagram, label each ray as a Roman numeral. Branches off those rays are capital letters (A, B, C) and in the outline and subbranches are 1,2,3.

To construct a formal outline using decimals directly from your Sun Diagram, label each ray as a number followed by a decimal. Branches off these rays are numbers with decimals (1.1.2).

SUCCESS DEPENDS ON GOOD ORGANIZATION

Whether we are coaching new writers on a one-to-one basis or teaching a writing workshop with more than twenty students, we have found that these 10 steps and the Sun Diagram have become the most useful organizing tools for our writers. Organizing is a very difficult skill for many new writers, yet organizing well is crucial to the success of an article and to success in publishing.

New writers consistently produce an organized manuscript using this process. They find the writing flowing more freely when they use these steps. Now you have done the hardest work and you are ready to write. But one more time . . . wait. Check your idea with an editor before you write, so you can write the article the journal wants to publish. The next chapter addresses communicating with editors.

EXERCISE

Complete the ten steps to organize the content of your manuscript.

REFERENCES

Adams, J. E. (1979). *Conceptual blockbusting.* New York: W. W. Norton.

Brusaw, C. T., Alred, G. J., & Oliu, W. E. (1993). *Handbook of technical writing.* New York: St. Martin's Press.

Burkhalter, P. K. (1976). So you want to write! *Supervisor Nurse, 7*(6), 54–56.

Clutter, P., Easter, A., Gloe, D., & Kiner, R. (1994). Help! She's been shot. *RN, 57*(9), 45–50.

Dennis, K. E., & Prescott, P. A. (1985). Florence Nightingale: Yesterday, today, and tomorrow. *Advances in Nursing Science, 7*(2), 66–81.

Dowdney, D. L. (1984). For professional advancement: Your resume. *Nursing Management, 15*(8), 13–14.

Fanning, T., & Fanning, R. (1979). *Get it all done and still be human.* New York: Ballantine Books.

Fawcett, H., Ferdinand, S., & Rockley, A. (1993). The design draft—Organizing information. In C. N. Barnum & S. Carliner (Eds.), *Techniques for technical communications.* New York: Macmillan.

Flower, L. (1985). *Problem-solving strategies for writing.* New York: Harcourt Brace Jovanovich.

Horn, R. E. (1989). *Mapping hypertext.* Lexington, MA: Lexington Institute.

Johnson, S. H. (1982). Developing an article using the nursing model. *Dimensions of Critical Care Nursing, 1*(1), 58.

Jones, I. H. (1983, August 24). Getting into writing. *Nursing Mirror, 15*(8), 46–47.

Mack, K., & Skjei, E. (1979). *Overcoming writing blocks.* Los Angeles: J. P. Tarcher.

McMillan, W. I. (1985). 10 steps to creativity. *Nursing Success Today, 2*(3), 14–15.

Michaelson, H. B. (1990). *How to write and publish engineering papers and reports.* Phoenix, Oryx Press.

Morra, M. E. (1984). How to plan and carry out your poster session. *Oncology Nursing Forum, 11*(2), 52–57.

Polit, D. F., & Hungler, B. P. (1983). *Nursing research principles and methods*. Philadelphia: J. B. Lippincott.

Rico, G. L. (1983). *Writing the natural way*. Los Angeles: J. P. Tarcher.

Sheridan, D. R., & Spector, D. (1984). Assessing current management development needs. *Stanford Nurse, 6*(3), 11–13.

Southby, J. R. (1981). Preparing a written research report. *AORN Journal, 33*(4), 719.

Treece, E. W., & Treece, J. W., Jr. (1973). *Elements of research in nursing*. St. Louis: C. V. Mosby.

VanAlstyne, J. S., & Maddison, G. R. (1994). *Professional & technical writing strategies*. Englewood Cliffs, NJ: Prentice-Hall.

Whalen, E. (1994). Formal outlining for writers and editors. In Minick, P., (Ed.), *Biomedical communication: Selected AMWA workshops*. Bethesda, MD: American Medical Writers Association.

Wheeler, C. E. (1985). *The American Journal of Nursing* and the socialization of a profession 1900–1920. *Advances in Nursing Science, 7*(2), 20–34.

Yura, H., & Walsh, M. B. (1978). *The nursing process*. New York: Appleton-Century-Crofts.

7

Communicate with Editors

Open communication with editors is essential to having your manuscripts accepted for publication. Frequently nursing journal editors ask writers to prepare articles for their publications. Manuscripts that are written because of editors' requests are called "solicited manuscripts."

We asked nursing journal editors how they determine appropriate authors from whom they solicit manuscripts. Most editors replied that they looked for evidence of expertise and knowledge in particular areas. That is, they solicited manuscripts from leaders in the field who were nationally known experts in the topic area. Editors solicited articles from previously published authors who had published on the topic; they also solicited articles from individuals who gave speeches at national nursing conferences, seminars, workshops, and other professional meetings.

In addition, editors solicited articles based on recommendations from editorial board members and advisors, supervisors in various institutions, state nursing associations, and contacts in the health care field. Editors indicated they looked for nurses performing research in a particular area and for persons who were good writers.

Sometimes editors solicited manuscripts from groups that submitted letters or news releases about nursing activities. Editors also gave assignments to writers who sent them promising resumes and clips of previously published materials. Finally, editors commented that they looked for writers with experience, education, and enthusiasm.

METHODS OF INITIATING CONTACT WITH EDITORS

Usually editors do not make the initial contact—writers do. We asked nurse writers how they initiated contact for their first article. Those asked indicated that they used one or a combination of the following three methods to contact editors: sending a query letter; sending the completed manuscript; or telephoning the editor.

We also asked selected nurse authors in our survey how they made the initial contact with the editor of their first published article. Their responses indicated a variety of methods:

GENROSE J. ALFANO: I just submitted the article.

IRENE M. BOBAK: The editor contacted me.

LUTHER CHRISTMAN: The editor was in the audience when I gave the paper and solicited the manuscript.

DONNA DIERS: I just sent in the manuscript.

SR. ROSEMARY DONLEY: I sent the article and letter.

MARGARET L. MCCLURE: The journal approached me and asked me to write the article.

BARBARA STEVENS BARNUM: I simply sent my completed article with a cover letter.

DUANE D. WALKER: I sent a letter and followed up with a phone call.

HELEN YURA: By letter at the suggestion of my teacher.

MARY LLOYD ZUSY: I wrote a query letter to the editor describing what I intended to write and why I thought they would be interested in it.

From your initial idea through the process of developing and publishing your manuscript, you and your editor will have a series of communications. For a quality article, you and your editor need to work together to produce a product of value to the journal's readership. Listen openly and nondefensively to editors' suggestions because editors have a different perspective from yours. In addition, they make the final publication decisions.

An example of working together might be something like this: You send a query letter to the editor of *The Nurse* describing your topic, patient classification, and why it is appropriate for this publication. The editor responds that "an article is in press on using patient classification systems to enhance cost containment which covers. . ." The editor asks you how your article will be different. The editor may have some specific suggestions about how you might make it different. Consider these ideas and change your manuscript. Most nursing journal editors who offer suggestions are trying to help you get your article published; their feedback may give you specific ideas.

Use the editor's feedback to match your manuscript to specific editorial/publication needs or redefine your market. Our strong advice to you is to take the editor's suggestions. Either way, let editors know that you appreciate their ideas and inform them of what you have decided to do. The communication between editor and writer continues from query through editing and publication. Give feedback to the editor that you heard the message. Send your decision. This process should continue through editing and publication. Without this open two-way communication between you and an editor, your chances of publication diminish.

When you write an article or book manuscript, you may work with several editors, including the acquisitions editor, developmental editor, and the production editor. By knowing what each editor is responsible for, you will be able to communicate with the right person when you have a question or need help with your manuscript (Johnson, 1993).

Nursing journals are beginning to post their writer's guidelines on the Internet. We downloaded the following information from *The Journal of Nursing Jocularity* directly from the Internet via CompuServe. The journal's posting included a questionnaire, a checklist for artists and the following checklist for authors. It also included suggestions and ideas for humorous material and descriptions of the needs for various departments and fillers.

JOURNAL OF NURSING JOCULARITY'S WRITER'S GUIDELINES

Journal of Nursing Jocularity
P. O. Box 40416
Mesa, AZ 85274
Phone 602–835–6165
FAX 602–835–6165
CompuServe Address: Doug Fletcher 73314,3032
Internet Address: INTERNET:73314.3032@compuserve.com

Dear Colleague:

The Journal of Nursing Jocularity, the humor magazine for nurses, is looking for quality stories and artwork. We assume you have seen a copy of the JNJ, and know the type of material we use. If you would like a sample copy of the JNJ please send a $3.00 check or money order. If you are interested in contributing material to the magazine, fill out the enclosed questionnaire (page 2) and return it to us. This will put you on our mailing list for updates on the JNJ's progress.

Unlike most other nursing journals, the Journal of Nursing Jocularity will pay contributors upon publication. For manuscripts we pay 2 cents per printed word (average page in JNJ is 400–500 words). A 1000 word story would pay $20. For artwork we pay $5 to $25 per illustration or cartoon, according to work involved and perceived value. Average payment for a cartoon is $10. We pay $100 for a cover illustration. See page 4 for information about doing a cover illustration.

All material submitted will be considered for publication. We will mail you a postcard on receipt of the manuscript or artwork to let you know that it was received. It can take one to three months to determine if a submission will be used, depending on when we receive it in our publishing cycle. We plan the JNJ nine to twelve months in advance, so it can take a year or more before an accepted story is actually printed.

Once material is accepted for publication in the JNJ, the journal will hold all magazine and reprint rights (see sample Publishing Agreement). With the popularity of the humor in the Journal of Nursing Jocularity, we are receiving frequent requests from hospitals, nursing schools and health organizations to reprint material from the JNJ. We would like to be able to freely grant permission to these organizations and encourage the spread of humor. We DO NOT ask for any reimbursement for reprint permission. If you don't agree with this publishing agreement, please contact us, and we can determine an arrangement that will work for both of us. Prior to publication, we will send you a publishing agreement to sign and return. The publishing agreement will include the amount that we will pay for the piece. Also included in this packet is a "Check List." Please use this to insure you are sending the submission in the proper format.

We look forward to seeing your work.

Yours in jocularity,

Doug Fletcher, RN
Publisher

Fran London, MS, RN
Editor

P.S. Feel free to make copies of this file for friends interested in submitting work to the JNJ.

ABOUT SENDING WORK ON FLOPPY DISK
- Manuscripts sent on computer disk can be sent in any of the following formats: IBM compatible, 5-1/4" or 3-1/2", and Mac 3-1/2." We should be able to convert from most word processors. Please specify story name, computer type and word processor on the labeled disk.
- Enclosed a self addressed, stamped envelope with adequate postage if you want a disk in return.

ABOUT SENDING WORK VIA COMPUSERVE
Manuscripts may be submitted to the JNJ via CompuServe at address 73314,3032. It must include title page and article body as described above. It can be sent in any

of the formats described in the "Floppy Disk" paragraph above. After it is received, most correspondence will be via snail mail (U.S. postal service).

Reprinted with permission from *Journal of Nursing Jocularity*, Writer's Guidelines.

PLANNING YOUR QUERY LETTERS

Query letters introduce you and your manuscript idea to an editor. Effective query letters attract the editor's interest, show that you are qualified to write the manuscript, indicate that you understand the journal's target audience, and serve as an example of your ability to write clearly. Your query letter is a sample of how you think and write. In addition, your query letter describes your topic, why readers will want to know about it, and why the editor should consider it for publication. Well-written query letters reveal your ability to write clearly and succinctly.

Writing a query letter saves you time because it allows you to explore an editor's interest in your topic before you write the article; thus, you can adapt what you are writing to the editor's suggestions. Then you can write your manuscript according to a specified length and meet the needs of the publication's target audience. When editors give your query a "go ahead," they expect your manuscript; they will probably publish it if it meets their standards and expectations. The query reserves a place for your story.

Query letters also save you time because you discover when editors would not be interested in your manuscript before you have invested your time writing. Query letters keep you from wasting valuable time writing a manuscript that has little possibility of publication. Query letters also save you time in finding the "right" journal for your article because you can mail several letters simultaneously to different journals. (Manuscripts should be mailed to only one journal at a time). Query letters save postage costs too because they cost less to send than mailing complete manuscripts. In addition, most editors of nursing and health care journals expect queries rather than complete manuscripts.

Whenever you have a choice, send a query letter prior to writing the article. Marta Vivas (1982) wrote, "It is generally considered advisable to query a journal regarding a proposed article first, before sending in an unsolicited manuscript" (p. 484). The query letter gives you contact with the editor and can save possible rejection later. It allows you to discover what is required editorially, and what slant the editor wishes to emphasize.

Although you do not have to write the article before sending the query, you do need to spend some time thinking, planning, and organizing your article. You need to do some library searching for your target market, and perhaps some researching on the content. Do just enough work to organize your thoughts so you can sell your article.

In query letters, editors like to hear why their target market would be interested in your article. Be specific and avoid cliches. Believe in what you sell. Salespeople say that you can only sell something in which you believe. There is no better way to sell something than to offer it to someone who is looking for just that item to buy. Thus, explain why the readers of that journal would be interested in reading whatever you are writing. Journal editors told us they like to hear from authors who write well, who are enthusiastic, and who have great interest in the topic. If you do not believe a particular publication's audience will be interested in your article, look for the right market—a journal whose readers need to know what you have to say.

If ten articles have recently appeared on your topic, editors will not be interested in one more article on the same topic unless you have a unique slant appropriate to their specific market. Do your homework. Find out which editors want your manuscript.

In our survey of randomly selected nurse authors (Sheridan and Dowdney, 1984), those who used query letters to initiate contact with an editor said:

- "I sent a query letter. The editors asked to see my manuscript. After it was reviewed, they returned it to me for revision."
- "I sent a query letter that indicated my interest. My query received a positive response, so I sent the article."
- "I sent a query. It was a lengthy process because it took them three months to tell me they were interested in my article. I sent the manuscript four months later. They sent it back with suggestions for revision. Then the airlines lost the manuscript with the baggage. The editors sent me a photocopy so that I could make changes."
- "I sent a query letter. It took one year for the review and revisions before the manuscript was published."
- "I received a positive response to my query letter. The article was printed within a few months. Then the editors solicited a second article a few months later."
- "I wrote a query letter after I received a list of upcoming journal topics. They telephoned me about interest in the content and wanted to expand the article to encompass an entire 'on the scenes' focus for our institution. As a result, others wrote an additional article to complete the project. I received one review of the total article with only minor editing revisions."

Because editors are bombarded with completed manuscripts and query letters, your initial contact is extremely important. The old saying "You only have one chance to make a good first impression" is true for each manuscript or query letter you send to each editor.

To enhance your chance of sparking editorial interest, try to understand what editors need and want. Then send it to them. "Most editors (70% or more) are primarily responsible for establishing editorial policy; planning journal content; recruiting and working with reviewers and editorial advisors; corresponding and working with authors; initial manuscript reading; design and layout; soliciting manuscripts; and substantive editing" (Binger, 1982, p. 263). Thus, communicating with editors is vital for your manuscript's publication because editors also select reviewers who will evaluate your manuscript for publication.

You may initiate contact with editors before you write your manuscript by sending query letters, by telephoning, or by meeting editors at conferences and professional events. Many nursing journal editors prefer receiving a query letter rather than an unsolicited manuscript. Yet, there are editors who prefer to receive the manuscript. A few even prefer telephone calls or an outline.

We asked 47 nursing journal editors what type of initial contact they preferred. Twenty-three journal editors preferred query letters, eighteen preferred manuscripts, four preferred a telephone inquiry, and two preferred written outlines. Today, many editors are open to query letters being faxed and manuscripts sent on disk.

If you send an unsolicited manuscript to an editor who prefers receiving a query letter, the editor will probably have an unfavorable response to the manuscript. Worse yet, handwritten manuscripts and manuscripts with grammatical, spelling, or punctuation errors almost guarantee instant rejection because better quality is expected from a professional. Manuscripts are rarely coveted enough to overcome poor work quality and scholarship.

Be sure to read and follow editorial guidelines, which are often stated inside or near the journal's cover. They are also available without charge from the nursing journal editors. Straying from guidelines can hinder your chances of rousing the editor's interest, especially when you are submitting a manuscript as your initial contact.

Before You Send a Query Letter

Before you send a query letter, be sure you have completed the earlier steps of the Writing Process, especially investigating the editorial needs of specific journals and gathering enough material to sound authoritative. In addition, you should have your material well organized with a completed Writing Plan,

Target Journal Analysis Forms for each possible target, traditional outline or detailed Sun Diagram, and preliminary contacts with interviewees if your topic involves interviews and a strong lead (explained later in this chapter).

What to Include in a Query Letter

Begin your query letter with a strong "lead" or a "hook" that will attract the editor's attention and convince the editor that the publication's readers will be interested in your topic. Your first paragraph can be the same as your article's lead. For example, in the article "For Professional Advancement: Your Resume," the author began her query, "An effective resume is one of a nurse's most valuable tools for professional advancement." This was later the first sentence in her article published by *Nursing Management* (Dowdney, 1984).

Next, your query should establish your expertise—both expertise in writing (if any) and experience with the article's subject matter. Include any titles of previously published articles and where they were published. Explain your expertise or special work that prepared you for writing this manuscript, such as a course in economics or clinical work in the field. Mention your academic background if it reveals your special insights into the topic, or if you are writing to individuals in academic settings. Even if you attach a resume, do not skip this paragraph in the query letter. Editors want to be able to see why you are qualified to write this article without paging through your resume to try to figure it out.

The sources or resources you will use may be worth sharing. Perhaps you have forms created as part of a system you have developed at work. If you will be interviewing people, indicate the names, expertise (titles, etc.) of the interviewees, and their willingness to be interviewed. Editors need to know how you will obtain your facts and how accurate they will be. Editors also may want to recommend additional resources.

Also include in the query letter when the article will be ready, the length of the article, and whether you plan to include illustrative materials in the article. Sometimes, in addition to a query letter, editors may like to see "tearsheets," which are copies of your previously published articles. If you have tearsheets that reveal your expertise in the area, if your articles have appeared in a prestigious publication, or if they reveal your best writing, send them.

Query Letter Style

Use the style that the publication uses. If it uses a formal style, imitate it. On the other hand, if the publication uses a conversational style, use that in your query letter. Begin positively, rather than with phrases such as "Although I have not written anything since high school. . .". If you have not been published before, do not address the issue at all.

Be sure to give some specific details or facts rather than vague generalities. For example, do not say you work in the delivery room and want to write an article on nursing students. Rather, state that you have 6 years of experience instructing student nurses during their clinical experience in perinatal nursing and have found some effective measures for helping them deal with crises. Give information about both authors if writing together, especially if it shows combined expertise in relation to the topic. For example, the authors of "Bone Marrow Transplantation: An Overview and Comparison of Autologous, Syngeneic, and Allogeneic Treatment Modalities" include a pediatric clinical/pharmacology research nurse, a pediatric oncology outpatient clinical nurse, and an oncology infectious disease research nurse (Cogliano-Shutta, Broda, & Gress, 1985).

Another example of combined expertise is the article by coauthors Chinn and Wheeler, who wrote "Feminism and Nursing" (1985). One author is a nursing professor; the other, also a nurse, is President of Margaret's Daughters, a feminist group.

Keep your sentences to a 20-word or less average, and use variety in your sentence construction. Be brief and clear. Inquire about only one manuscript idea in each query letter.

Developing the Query Letter

You can organize the elements of a query letter on a Sun Diagram. Write your working title in the center, and add a minimum of four rays. On one ray, place elements of your lead. On another ray, address the resources and sources you will use for your article. Such resources could be research studies, interviews, work performed on a task force, literature review, or a case study experience. On another ray, let the editor know why you should write this manuscript. Indicating writing and/or clinical expertise in the area. The fourth ray is for logistics such as how soon you could have a completed article to the editor and in how many words. Each ray will probably develop into a paragraph or two depending on your topic. Figure 7.1 presents a model Sun Diagram for a query letter.

To illustrate the query letter, the actual query letter Donna Dowdney used is presented in Figure 7.2. The article that resulted from the query letter appeared in *Nursing Management* in August, 1984. The Sun Diagram in Figure 7.3 illustrates the above query letter.

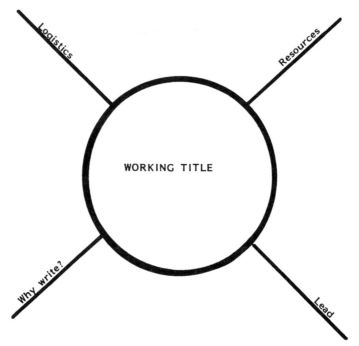

Figure 7.1. Sun Diagram for a query letter (Dowdney & Sheridan © 1982).

The Lead

Remember, begin your query letter with your strong lead or "hook" to entice the editor to read your letter. This same lead can later be used to begin your article. A strong opening introduces the general theme of the article and draws the reader to continue reading the article.

Your lead paragraph can also summarize your article's main idea and present the style and viewpoint in which you write the article. The following paragraphs should include enough facts and anecdotes to convince the editor of the article's accuracy and flavor. Since the first sentence of your query can often be the first sentence of your article, consider the following types of lead sentences that could open query letters: newsworthy information, fact, quotation, question, shocking statement, typical example, history, definition, future orientation, statistics, or commonly acknowledged problem.

Below are examples of lead sentences. Do they hook you? Do you want to know more?

Dear Editor:

An effective resume is one of a nurse's most valuable tools for professional advancement. With it, the nurse can seize opportunities as they present themselves; without it, the nurse may watch opportunities disappear before there is time for the resume to be assembled.

An effective resume skillfully and concisely presents the nurse's academic and professional background while revealing skills and knowledge that may be used in the new opportunity or setting. A poorly prepared resume merely states dates and places, but it does not show the scope of the responsibility or highlight the expertise obtained in previous settings.

As Director of Writing Enterprises International, I have prepared hundreds of resumes, curriculum vitae, and dossiers for professionals, many in the field of nursing. From the expertise gained through preparing these resumes, I am writing a 2,000 word article on resumes for nurses. The article will deal with the following areas: what information to include in a professional resume, how to slant the resume to highlight skills needed in particular positions, methods of organization, and formats. I have also taught classes in communications in a medical setting at Stanford University Medical Center. Currently I am teaching seminars there in Writing for Professional Publication in Nursing.

My feature articles have appeared in diverse publications including *California Highway Patrolman*, *Glass Digest*, and *Decision*. In August 1982, my article on Executive Resumes will appear in *Accent Magazine*. Currently I serve as President of the Palo Alto Branch of the National League of American Pen Women, and I am a member of California Writers Club and the American Business Communications Association. I am also a contributing editor to *Writers Connection*.

Please let me know if you would like me to send you my article, "Resumes for Nurses." Also let me know if you would be interested in other articles related to "Writing for Publication in Nursing." I would be glad to develop such articles to your specifications.

Sincerely,

Donna Lee Dowdney

Figure 7.2. A query letter that worked (© 1982 Dowdney).

Fact. In *Pediatric Nursing*, Hanrahan, Kleiber, and Fagan began: "While the efficacy of heparin versus saline has been extensively studied in adults, [10 cites are listed] . . . until very recently studies were lacking in the pediatric population (1994, p. 549).

Quotation. In an article on planning entitled "It Matters Which Way You Go: Facilitating Planning" that appeared in *Staff Development Insider*, a quotation began the column:

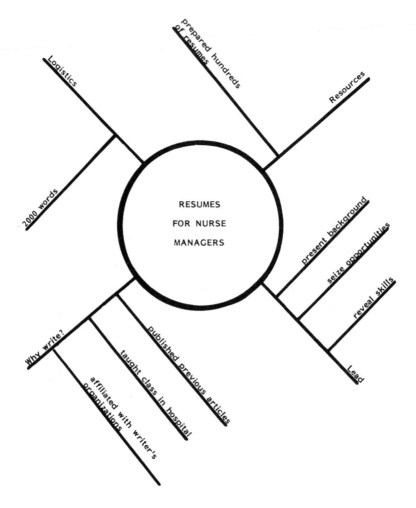

Figure 7.3. Sun Diagram for specific query letter (Dowdney © 1982).

In Lewis Carroll's *Alice's Adventures in Wonderland*. Alice asked the Cheshire Cat, "Would you please tell me which way I ought to go from here?" The cat answered, "That depends a good deal on where you want to get to." "I don't care much where." said Alice. To which the cat retorted 'then it doesn't much matter which way you go.' (Sheridan, 1994, p. 1).

Question.   Mary A. Alexander, in "Evaluating the Behavioral Objectives" (1985, p. 63) began her article with a series of questions: "Behavioral objectives are acknowledged to be an integral part of educational evaluation, but how can we evaluate the objectives themselves? How can we determine whether or not educational programs are really giving participants what they want? And how can we provide a means for participants to evaluate the fulfillment of a program's objectives?"

Shocking Statement. "A poster widely displayed by Research! America provides the following alert: Warning: Insufficient Medical Research Can Be Hazardous To Your Health" begins an article explaining why the American Academy of Nursing joined Research! America (Pender, 1993, p. 152). Even more shocking was the opener: "In the time it takes you to read this article, three women in the United States will develop breast cancer," began Sandra J. Eich's article, "Promising Early Breast Cancer Treatment— Without Mastectomy" (1985, p. 51).

Typical Example. "A 24-year-primigravida was admitted at 41 weeks with spontaneous rupture of the membranes. Labour was augmented with oxytocin, and epidural anaesthesia was administered. After 20 hours, lower segment caesarean section was performed because of failure to progress in the first stage of labour. The patient was irritable, rather confused and felt dizzy." Thus began R. Haloob's article, "Oxytocin Induced Hyponatremia" (1984, p. 104).

History. An article in *Nurse Educator* on tribal education began: "America's mainstream colleges have enrolled Native American students for more than 350 years, but the goal was almost always assimilation, seldom the enhancement of the American Indian students or the well-being of their tribes. Tribal colleges, in sharp contrast, have demonstrated over the last 25 years that cultural strengthening, not assimilation, are supportive and nurturing to Native American students (Demarest & Sokoloff, 1994, p. 32).

Definition. A definition of perception began the article "Perceptual Dysfunction: Nursing Assessment and Management" (Wyness, 1985): "Perception is the ability to receive input from the senses and to interpret and correlate this input in a meaningful way" (p. 105).

Personal Interest. In order to motivate the staff nurse, this article begins: "Although you already know that the Joint Commission on Accreditation of Health Care Organizations (JCAHO) has revised its survey process, you may still be wondering how this will affect you. The answer is: directly" (Moore-Greenlaw, & Hurley, 1994, p. 31).

Statistics.   Statistical information began Jane Sharber's article on "Oxygen Radicals and Calcium Ion Flux: Role in Reperfusion Injury Following AMI" (1994, p. 256): "Acute myocardial infarction (AMI) disease secondary to coronary artery disease (CAD) remains the leading cause of death in the United States. The American Heart Association estimated 1,500,000 incidences of AMI, with more than 500,000 fatalities for 1991."

Commonly Acknowledged Problem.

Domestic violence is now recognized as a national health problem, as well as a community, family, and partner problem . . . There is general agreement by experts in the field of domestic violence that almost all partner abuse is inflicted by men against women (95%) and that partner abuse crosses all social, cultural, racial, economic and educational lines (U.S. Department of Health and Human Services, 1990. Attala, Oetker, & McSweeney, 1995, pp. 17–24)

This opener set up an article to deal with this commonly acknowledged problem.

Story.   "Hurry, hurry! the little girl said to herself. "The sun's almost down and I've got to get home before it gets dark." Murray began her article in AJN (1993, p. 36) relating one nurse's personal experience with diabetic neuropathy.

What Does Not Go into a Query Letter

Now, a few don'ts about the query letter. Even if you are publishing to attain tenure, do not tell the editor that your career and reputation are staked on your manuscript's publication! Do not begin with a negative thought such as, "Although your journal has not dealt with this issue . . .". Do not use sales/advertising hype about the manuscript such as, "This is the greatest article you'll ever see." Do not give too much information in the query letter; it is not the place to write your whole article, but rather to attract attention and whet the appetite for the rest of the article. Do not mention a fee desired because nursing journals usually do not pay one. You may ask if a fee is paid, but that is not a good idea if you are a new writer. Do not ask for advice or other marketing sources. Do not include more than one article idea in a query letter.

TYPING AND SENDING YOUR QUERY LETTER

Type your query letter as one single-spaced page. Use at least one-inch margins and make a photocopy for your files. Be sure to include your name and return address. Send your letter to the current editor. You can find the editor's name by looking at the editor's box of a current issue or by checking resources such as *Writer's Market, Literary Market Place,* or *Business Publication Rates and Data.* Enclose a self-addressed, stamped envelope (SASE), a list of previously published articles, and your resume if you wish to document your expertise.

Checklist for the Query Letter

- Did you send the letter to a specific editor?
- Did you describe your topic well enough so that editors will see its importance to the journal's readers?
- Did you show how you will approach the topic (how-to, personal experience, survey, research)?
- Did you show your article's benefits to the readers—the reasons why it is important?
- Did you use a strong lead that compels the editor to want to see your article?
- Did your title convey the essence of your manuscript?
- Did you convince the editor that you are familiar with the journal's needs, format, readership, editorial policies, and style as reflected in recent issues?
- Did you indicate the sources of information you will use in preparing the article?
- Did you show that your article is current and timely by tying the article into a new discovery, a news event, or recently released statistics?
- Did you convey your enthusiasm for the topic and manuscript?
- Did you show what your expertise and qualifications are for writing the article?
- Did you write concisely and convincingly so that it serves as a sample of the way you think and write?
- Did you use good grammar, spelling, and punctuation?
- Did you organize your query so that it is clear?
- Did you urge the editor to take action?
- Does your query reveal your professionalism in tone and style?
- Did you enclose a stamped, addressed return envelope?
- Did you keep an accurate record of when, where, and to whom you sent the query letter?
- Did you keep a photocopy for your files?

Multiple Query Letters

You can send multiple query letters, but not manuscripts, to several different publications simultaneously. In fact, it is a good idea to have several query letters in the mail at all times. Gordon Burgett, author of *The Query Book,* (1980) *Query Letters—Cover Letters: How They Sell Your Writing* (1986); and *The Writer's Guide to Query Letters and Cover Letters* (1991) tries to keep many queries alive at a time, knowing that about a third will bring first-response "go-aheads."

If you use a word processor or a computer with a word-processing program, you can easily prepare several queries using the same paragraphs about your article, your qualifications, and available photographs. You can change the journal, editor, and address, and write your query specifically to deal with the needs of that particular editor and journal. You can plan your letters to go out in batches using word processing equipment to turn out many query letters at one time (Zobel, 1992)

RESPONSES TO QUERY LETTERS

Editors of nursing and health care journals usually take 2 to 6 weeks to respond to query letters. You will probably receive one of the following three responses to your query letter:

- Positive "acceptance letter": An interest in the manuscript.
- Negative "rejection slip": No interest in the manuscript.
- No response (ambiguous): May or may not be interested in the manuscript.

Acceptance

Although an editor may show interest in your article, this does not guarantee your manuscript's publication. A positive response to a query is given in good faith that the writer will send a quality manuscript in the publication's format at the agreed-upon time.

When you receive an acceptance letter, send a brief letter of confirmation to the editor. Indicate the date on which you will send the manuscript. React to any editorial recommendations, and confirm any changes the editor suggested—unless you cannot accept them. If you cannot accept the editor's recommendations, suggest an alternative. Recognize the editor's perspective. New authors tend to have more difficulty than experienced ones in accepting editorial suggestions. One experienced author said she really appreciated editor's suggestions because the time the editor took to offer suggestions had great payoffs. Often editor's ideas help to focus the material and direct it to the journals' need and to the readers' interests. This is not to suggest that you change your values or present something in which you do not believe. An editor may suggest changes such as including nursing implications, asking you to explain why something is a problem for others (generalize), or taking a more educational perspective.

Editors know their journals and readers well. If you disagree with an editor's judgment, you risk not being published for what you might not realize until later is naivete on your part. Consider editors' suggestions with an open mind.

Review your Writing Plan. Adjust the dates on your time line, beginning with the date you receive your acceptance letter. Write your tasks on a calendar. The earlier rough outline you completed puts you well into the writing process for your article. Adjust the diagram to meet the editor's recommendations, schedule a trip to the library for any missing data, then proceed to the next step of this process—writing the manuscript (Chapter 8).

Rejection

In our survey of selected nurse authors, we asked, "Have your manuscripts/query letters ever been rejected? If yes, what did you do with the rejected manuscripts/query letters?" The authors replied:

GENROSE J. ALFANO: Yes. Sometimes I re-wrote. Sometimes I submitted it to another journal. Sometimes I let it be!

SARAH E. ARCHER: Yes. I sent them to other journals. Occasionally I forgot the whole thing.

BARBARA J. BROWN: Yes. I tried again using a more diverse and creative approach.

DOROTHY J. DEL BUENO: Yes. Only 1 out of 55—and I had it published somewhere else after re-working it.

RHEBA DE TORNYAY: Yes. Heaven's yes. I've had manuscripts rejected! Some I tossed away. Others, I submitted to another journal.

DONNA DIERS: Yes. Two manuscripts were rejected. One deserved it, and I pitched it. The other didn't, so I used it for teaching purposes. (It was rejected because the journal was a year behind in publishing and had to clear out its files.)

VERNICE FERGUSON: Yes. No further pursuits. I served as the second of two authors. The manuscript was not the best.

LOUCINE M. HUCKABAY: Yes. I re-wrote it and re-submitted it to the same journal and it was accepted. Some I sent to another nursing journal and they were accepted.

MARGARET L. MCCLURE: Yes. By the time the NLN (League Exchange) rejected the manuscript, the material was too old to use.

M. JANICE NELSON: Yes. I wrote back and requested more specific information.

BARBARA STEVENS BARNUM: Yes. I had one manuscript rejected once because the publisher felt that my recommendations would decrease his book sales. I just scrapped the article.

MARGRETTA M. STYLES: Yes. I used their recommendations as a basis for revising the manuscript. I have had one paper rejected twice and am in the process of re-writing again.

DUANE D. WALKER: Yes. I submitted it to a different journal.

HELEN YURA: Yes and no. I sought an alternative source for publishing and was successful.

MARY LLOYD ZUSY: Yes. Ultimately, I gave up on one of them after offering it to several journals.

When editors reject manuscripts, they often send "rejection sips" or letters indicating reasons for rejection. Others send personal letters including reasons for the rejection; still others send a standard "not interested" form letter back to you. Such form letters often do not let you know why the editor rejected your article; they do not give you any clues about whether to pursue other markets, change the manuscript, or try a different article altogether.

Lawrence Block discussed rejection slips as raising questions such as "What is one to make of the language of a publisher's rejection? What does 'Not right for us at present' mean? Why don't publishers say *exactly* what they mean once you know how to translate their remarks:

> When a publisher says your manuscript is not suitable at the present, that it's not quite right for his list, that it doesn't suit his current needs, it means one thing and one thing only.
>
> It means he doesn't want to publish it.
>
> And that, when you come right down to it, is all he has to say and all you have to know. That he does not express himself more candidly testifies to his consideration for your feelings. Surely editors must yearn to put the matter more forcefully now and then. "This is garbage!" "I wouldn't line my parakeet's cage with these pages!"

Yet, as Block continued, "Editors rarely behave so brutally" (Block, 1983, p. 9).

Some editors send checklists that indicate the reason for rejection. Such checklists can help you because you can decide what to do next based on the editor's feedback, particularly if you receive more than one rejection of a similar query. Sometimes receiving a rejection has nothing to do with a manuscript's quality. For example:

- The editor may have a similar manuscript ready to be published or assigned to another writer.
- The journal may have recently published an article on the same topic.
- The topic may not be appropriate for the particular publication.
- The idea is too vague or general for the journal's readership.
- The journal is overstocked with articles for the present.

At other times, receiving a rejection results directly from the manuscript's quality. Examples of problems resulting in receiving rejections include:

- Lack of clarity
- Incorrect format—such as typing single-spaced with narrow margins
- Weak grammar
- Incorrect spelling
- Unclear tables/illustrations
- Lack of timeliness
- Lack of comprehensive coverage
- Lack of depth
- Inaccurate quotations
- Lack of significance to readers
- Unnumbered pages resulting in confused sequence
- Lack of generating enthusiastic attention by overuse of passive voice, jargon, etc.
- Lack of appropriateness
- Handwritten, photocopies, or difficult-to-read manuscripts using an unusual typeface (script, dot matrix, etc.)
- Changes scribbled in margins

"If your query letters are not getting any action, let your manuscript speak for itself. (If it in turn gets rejected 20 or 30 times without drawing any strong positive response, you might want to entertain the possibility that there's something wrong with it.)" (Block, 1983, p. 9).

In the June 1995 issue of *The Writer*, Gene Fehler (1995, pp. 20–22), author of articles, poems, and stories that have appeared in more than 300 publications, listed key factors for writers receiving rejections.

- You don't want to write; you just want to be published.
- You haven't read widely the kind of material you are trying to write.
- You haven't mastered writing techniques.
- You've been too easily discouraged.
- You haven't studied the market.

- You failed to follow up leads.
- You can't take criticism.
- Your writing is commonplace or lacks imaginative spark.
- Your query letters don't "sell" your idea.
- You don't revise before submitting your manuscript.
- You are too concerned with writing for a specific market.
- You haven't learned the editorial requirements of a specific market.
- You make excuses for not writing.
- You may not have the talent or skill to succeed at the level you'd envisioned.

Why Are Articles Rejected?

We asked nursing journal editors what their reasons were for rejecting manuscripts:

CRITICAL CARE NURSE: Lack of in-depth pathophysiology and poor organization.

TODAY'S OR NURSE: Inappropriate subject matter or covered sufficiently in prior issues, inappropriate format, and lack of depth.

HEART AND LUNG: Superficial/simplistic discussion, content errors, and poor paragraph construction.

JOURNAL OF NURSING ADMINISTRATION: Poorly written, content inappropriate for top-level nurse executives, superficial topic development.

NURSING RESEARCH: Poor research design.

THE CANADIAN NURSE: Not of interest/relevance to nurses/nursing. Also articles should generally have Canadian content.

JOURNAL OF EMERGENCY NURSING: Too basic, superficial, or textbook material rather than information which updates textbook knowledge. Too theoretical school papers (thesis type manuscripts with belabored implication for nursing). Too many nonclinical, psychosocial, and administration/education articles.

COMPUTERS IN HEALTH CARE: Not applicable to health care computerization as the tone is too commercial.

We have listed these general reasons in the editor's words because we believe knowing what the editors do not want will help you to avoid these pitfalls. Some reasons for rejection were less specific to particular journals (Dowdney & Sheridan, 1984):

- Too clinical, too much like a research paper.
- Topics not of interest to our readers, not enough nursing content.

- Insufficient development, inappropriate topics, inaccurate statistics, overpublished topics.
- Poor integration of nursing care with surgical technique.
- Content represents material already available in nursing literature, nursing aspects underdeveloped, content not at appropriate level for the audience.
- Poorly organized, little emphasis on nursing application, quality of study poor.
- Lack of reader interest, too clinical, and poorly written articles that are beyond repair.
- Nothing new in the content, of no practical use to our readers, too elementary for our readers, too poorly written to salvage.
- Too many similar articles already received, articles not detailed enough nor do they cover the subject adequately.
- Lack of imagination, poor spelling of medical terms (indicates lack of professionalism).
- Too broad, too poorly written, poor organization, too basic, grammatical errors.
- Poorly written or stale.
- Inappropriateness or irrelevance of topic.
- Inadequate documentation and/or literature review, poor research methodologies and/or applications.
- Not suitable material, poorly written, no new ideas or outlook.
- Poorly written or not appropriate subject.
- Subject area not of interest, style not upbeat or lively enough, sounds like a thesis or dissertation, theoretical rather than practical information.
- Story concept inappropriate for our editorial mix; we are already doing a similar piece.
- Based on insignificant research, narrow audience interest.
- Poorly written, poorly substantiated, not written for our audience.
- It does not fit our format or content needs.

Why Are Nursing Research Articles Rejected?

Nursing research articles may be rejected for reasons related to the research or the writing and, less often, the topic. Editors of *Nursing Research* told us their most common reason for rejecting a manuscript is poor research design. Other reasons given by research-oriented nursing journals for rejection include: the research is not valid, no new information is presented, or the research is poorly written.

> Many authors are uncertain what to do with all of the information they uncover in their research projects. Some try to put all of the information into one manuscript, thus making the manuscript 50 or more pages long with over 500 references and more than 10 illustrations. These thesis-style articles are usually rejected, or at best returned for revision

so states Johnson (1992, p. 1) in her article suggesting how to adapt theses to be publishable.

Nursing Research conducted a comprehensive review of all manuscripts declined from 1973 through 1975 (Carnegie, 1976). The manuscript problems found then are still common today: Editors rejected manuscripts because the manuscripts:

- made no contribution toward the advancement of scientific knowledge or research methodology;
- did not meet the criteria of a research project;
- were not consistent with the publication's purpose;
- were not organized or presented according to standards of scientific reporting;
- were weak in assumptions and limitations.

Editors also rejected manuscripts in which:

- conclusions were not based on presented data;
- literature was not reviewed sufficiently;
- inappropriate data collection methods were used;
- inappropriate statistical tests were used to analyze the data; and
- inadequate or out-of-date references were used.

An additional reason for rejection was the submission of manuscripts that had not been prepared specifically for publication in *Nursing Research*.

Florence Downs, Editor of *Nursing Research*, addressed the issue of rejection, sharing her perspective:

> Our rejection rate remains high. Every rejection letter contains a terse, enumerated critique. I apologize if the critiques are not couched in more niceties. However, time and reviewer availability preclude the construction of polished essays that might soften the blow. We do our best to be even-handed. Rumors to the contrary, we do not favor geographic regions or particular topics, designs, or methods. And we try to select the best work, regardless of the credentials of the author. If you believe we have erred in our evaluation of your work, please say so. We may not change our mind, but we will always reconsider the evaluation. (Downs, 1985, p. 3)

What to Do If You Receive a Rejection Letter

Receiving a rejection letter is a disappointing and sometimes painful experience. One nurse said, "Three years ago I sent a manuscript to a nursing journal. It was rejected. I haven't felt like taking it out of the drawer to look at it since then." Some writers take rejections personally: "My ideas aren't any good. I'll never be able to write anything."

In contrast, some writers react to rejection letters by increasing their determination and perseverance. *Writer's Encyclopedia* (Polking, 1983) recounts how Jesse Stuart's story "I Can Climb Higher Than You" was rejected 47 times before being accepted by and then winning the title of "Best Story of the Year" from one of the same magazines that had previously rejected it.

Peter Benchley sent the *New Yorker* between 50 and 100 stories before they bought one. Says Benchley: "You have to keep writing, keep submitting, and keep praying to the god of whimsy that some editor will respond favorably." By persisting, Peter Benchley eventually sold *Jaws, The Deep,* and *The Island* (Benchley, 1983, p. 24). In 1989, Benchley's *Rummies: A Novel* was published followed by *the Beast* in 1991. In 1994 *White Shark* was published.

If you receive a rejection slip, allow yourself enough time to think objectively about your manuscript. If the rejection is unjustified or unfair, ignore it. If the reasons for rejection are appropriate, make changes that correspond to specific criticisms.

Do not act on your first rejection letter if you mailed several query letters. Wait until other responses come back. If you receive three rejection letters after sending out three query letters, you have several alternatives. Comments from editors can provide valuable insights. If any say they would be interested "if you are willing to . . . ," treat this as an acceptance letter with editorial suggestions to be followed. If editors make other suggestions, try them. Perhaps an editor suggests using it in a "department" or as a letter to the editor or in an opinion section. Give this idea some serious consideration.

Try whatever the editor suggests and then query the editor again. If the letters were not encouraging, try another journal. You may even want to find some new markets, then select new target journals. Before you resubmit or submit a new query, ask a published colleague to read and critique your query and help you understand the reasons for rejection. Sometimes a fresh viewpoint can be helpful. Ask three colleagues to review the manuscript: one who understands the subject, one who has only limited knowledge of the subject, and one with a good writing background. Incorporate their comments into your revision.

When you ask colleagues for comments, do it in a way that allows them to tell you both positive and negative ideas. Otherwise, you may hear only positive comments. You might say, "I really need an honest critique to help me figure this out. Could you tell me what you think is right about it and what needs more work?" Or, "How can I write this better?" Then listen and take notes. Ask several colleagues, try to make the changes that are consistently suggested, and ask for other ideas that they think will help your manuscript.

What If I Receive No Response?

After 7 weeks, if you have not heard from an editor about your query, write or call to see if it was received. Ask when you can expect a response. If you write, attach a copy of your query in the event that it had been lost in the mail or otherwise misplaced.

After 3 months, a telephone call is appropriate. You have given an editor sufficient time to respond, and you need to know whether he or she is considering your manuscript. Always follow up because no response from nursing journal editors is unusual. Some editors send a postcard when they receive a manuscript. Often the postcard gives an approximate date on which you can expect a response.

In "Help! for Beginners Only," an article in *Writer's Digest*, Rose Adkins (1983, p. 71) responded to the following question from a reader: "If a query is rejected, can you go ahead and submit the manuscript to the editor who rejected the idea anyway?" She wrote: "While it is possible for an article to succeed where a query letter failed, it happens so rarely that trying that route isn't advisable." She went on to indicate that it would be better to polish the query and submit it to other magazines.

SENDING THE COMPLETE MANUSCRIPT

According to our survey, randomly selected nurse authors who sent complete manuscripts rather than query letters reported the following events that led to eventual publication:

- "I sent the manuscript. It was accepted and the editor sent a galley for my approval. I returned the galley, and the manuscript was published."
- "I sent the manuscript. It was accepted six weeks later by letter."
- "I sent the manuscript; it was returned for revisions. Then it was accepted for publication and was published two years later. I've been using query letters since then because they save time."

- "I sent the manuscript and followed-up with a telephone call. They liked the article, but couldn't use it for ten or eleven months. They asked if I'd mind waiting. I didn't mind, so they sent me a contract which I signed."
- "I sent the manuscript. It was accepted in eight months and published 2½ years later."
- "I sent the manuscript and received a letter asking me to convey copyright ownership."
- "I sent the manuscript and received a telephone contract of acceptance."
- "I sent the manuscript; the editor immediately agreed to publish the article."
- "I sent the manuscript and the article was accepted without revision almost immediately."
- "I sent the manuscript in 1968 and can't remember what happened!"
- "I sent the manuscript to the magazine. They called me in a week and told me they would review the article."
- "I sent the manuscript with a cover letter. They wrote me back and told me they had accepted the article. They instructed me to sign a release."
- "I sent the manuscript using the directions within the journal. Six weeks later they sent me a letter stating that my article had ben accepted."

TELEPHONE CONTACT

Usually you would not telephone an editor unless you have an article or story idea in which time is of the essence because of its newsworthiness. However, a few journal editors accept telephone queries as an initial contact. Before calling, look up the current editor's name in the journal.

Some randomly selected nurse authors we surveyed used the telephone successfully to discuss proposed articles with editors. They shared their experiences: "I telephoned the executive director of my professional association, who was also the editor." Another said, "I telephoned and then sent the manuscript." A third nurse author said, "I telephoned and sent a query letter. The editor accepted the content of the article, so I sent the manuscript. I waited over three years, then revised the article as the editor recommended."

Never call an editor without investing some time in the earlier stages of the Writing Process. Use the query letter Sun Diagram to organize your thoughts before you call. Be sure that you have reviewed a copy of the journal and have organized your content.

If you speak with an editor who gives you a "go ahead" over the telephone, follow up your conversation with a letter confirming your interest in writing the article you discussed over the telephone.

There are advantages to speaking directly with an editor over the telephone. You can quickly find out if the editor is interested in your article idea and receive additional ideas about the topic. The editor may have resource materials to send you or may know of current developments for you to incorporate into the article.

In addition, the editor may prefer a particular slant to the article and can give you that information over the telephone. For example, you may have brought together nurses in your specialty from several hospitals to solve a problem of mutual concern about a shared transport system. You would like to write an article on the problem and solution—i.e., an article about effective transport systems. You know it is a timely topic. Perhaps this journal is already planning an article on the topic (which often happens if a topic is timely.) The editor might suggest you develop the same article with a different slant. That is, the editor might be interested in an article about how you brought together nurses from several hospitals to collaboratively solve a problem of mutual concern. After you talk a few minutes, your new article idea begins to take shape. The former idea may still be an article for you to write for another journal.

On the telephone, you can also discuss your article to determine the appropriate style and target audience. You can also negotiate the time frame and any compensation.

PROFESSIONAL MEETINGS

Building a personal relationship with an editor is a good idea, particularly for a journal in your specialty. Most journals have regular writers whose work editors appreciate receiving. These regular writers send quality manuscripts on timely topics and can be counted on to come through whenever they make a commitment. You may be able to initiate a relationship at a professional meeting or convention. In fact, editors sometimes assign articles to writers they meet at professional meetings. If an editor gives your idea a positive response during a meeting, follow up with a letter indicating your understanding of the editor's interest.

When you write to an editor you have met or spoken with over the telephone, indicate any decisions reached during the conversation, the date on which the editor will receive the article, and any sample graphic or illustrative material. Your follow-up letter reminds the editor of your conversation and shows your serious intent to follow through with the article.

Your conversation with the editor can help you use the appropriate approach for the journal's readers. The editor may also ask you to write an abstract or summary and may suggest whether you should write in the first person or third person. In addition, the editor may let you know whether to include a sidebar. (A sidebar is a short feature that accompanies your article that may contain detailed information such as names and addresses, a checklist, or a related example that would disrupt your article's flow if not addressed separately.)

HOW EDITORS HELP

In our survey of randomly selected nurse authors, we asked how editors had helped the authors with their manuscripts and how editors could have been more helpful. Most responded that editors were quite supportive and that no additional help was needed.

- "The editors sent me the information and instructions I needed."
- "The editors gave me much encouragement to write another article."
- "The editors said that they liked my style."
- "The editors suggested areas to highlight."
- "The editors critique the content."
- "The editors suggested changes and specific revisions to be made."
- "The editors provided exquisite editing."
- "The editors revised for grammar and style."
- "The editors made substantive comments."
- "The editors put my article in the journal's format."
- "The editors sent back my rough draft with changes for my approval."
- "The editors requested additional information to make a few points more clear."
- "The editors called me long distance with questions about the manuscript."

A few survey respondents had suggestions on how editors could have been more helpful:

- "I wish they had edited more skillfully."
- "I wish they had contacted me during the time the article was awaiting publication."
- "I would have liked pay for my article!"
- "I would have liked an earlier acceptance notice and earlier publication date."

- "I wish they had spelled my name correctly. They were notified twice of the misspelling."
- "I would have liked a more timely response; it's very frustrating to wait and wait. I saw another journal publish an article on the same topic two months before my article."
- "I would have liked more communication about what they needed in regards to editing."

Finally, Hayes B. Jacobs (1984) indicated a few things that writers should not expect from editors:

- Writing instruction. "Editors have no time to teach you how to write; how to create work that they will then buy."
- Instant reports on submissions. "Your work, even if it has been solicited, is not the only thing on an editor's desk; he or she has many deadlines to worry about."
- Lengthy personal correspondence. "It's a business relationship; chitchat, in business, costs time and money, and an editor is paid to be conservative in both."
- Detailed marketing advice and strategies; advice on target journals. See the writer's guidelines and marketing books such as *Writer's Market*.
- Guarantees that your work will appear exactly as you wrote it. "Editors must be free to edit; factual errors, lack of clarity, excess, 'house style,' and personal references must be considered" (p. 8).

Working with an editor is rewarding. It has been our experience that nursing journal editors are, for the most part, fair and helpful. You can learn from editors' comments and editing. And working cooperatively with editors will enhance immeasurably your chances of publication. Now, with a positive response to a query in hand, you are ready to write . . . what an editor wants to publish. The three following chapters offer some helpful tips to turn out a quality manuscript in an efficient manner.

EXERCISES

1. Design a Sun Diagram for your query letter.
2. Write a lead (hook) for your article.
3. Write and send a query letter.

REFERENCES

Adkins, R. (1983, September). Help! for beginners only. *Writer's Digest,* 71.

Alexander, M. A. (1985). Evaluating the behavioral objectives. *Journal of Continuing Education in Nursing, 16*(2), 63.

Ames, D., & Madsen, N. (1981). Planing for change. *Nursing Administration Quarterly, 5*(2), 17–21.

Attala, J. M., Oetker, D., & McSweeney, M. (1995). Partner abuse against female nursing students. *Journal of Psychosocial Nursing, 33*(1), 17–24.

Benchley, P. (1983). *The complete guide to writing non-fiction.* Cincinnati: Writer's Digest.

Binger, J. L. (1982, April). Nursing journal editors. *Nursing Outlook, 30,* 263.

Block, L. (1983, December). Reflection slips. *Writer's Digest,* 9.

Burgett, G. (1980). *The query book.* Carpinteria, CA: Write to Sell.

Burgett, G. (1986). *Query letters—cover letters: How they sell your writing.* Carpinteria, CA: Write to Sell.

Burgett, G. (1991). The writer's guide to query letters and cover letters. Prima Publishers.

Business publication rates and data. (Monthly). Skokie, IL: Standard Rate and Data Service.

Carnegie, M. E. (1976). Rejection can be a challenge. *Nursing Research, 2*(3), 163.

Chinn, P., & Wheeler, C. E. (1985). Feminism and nursing. *Nursing Outlook, 33*(2), 74.

Cogliano-Shutta, N., Broda, E., & Gress, J. (1985). Bone marrow transplantation: An overview and comparison of autologous, syngeneic, and allogeneic treatment modalities. *Nursing Clinics of North America, 20*(1), 49.

DeJoseph, J., & O'Riordan, E. (1981). Claiming power: A strategy for change. *Nursing Administration Quarterly, 5*(2), 24–26.

Demarest, D. J., & Sokoloff, J. (1994). Tribal education: Reflections from the Pine Ridge Indian reservation. *Nurse Educator, 19*(4), 32–35.

Dowdney, D. L. (1984). For professional advancement: Your resume. *Nursing Management, 15*(8), 13–14.

Dowdney, D. L., & Sheridan, D. R. (1984). Survey of nursing and healthcare journal editors. Unpublished work.

Downs, F. S. (1985). News from the fourth estate. *Nursing Research, 34*(1), 3.

Eich, S. J. (1985, February). Promising early breast cancer treatment—without mastectomy. *Cancer Nursing, 8*(1), 51.

Fehler, G. (1995, June). Fourteen reasons for rejection: *The Writer,* 20–22.

Fletcher, D., & London, F. (1995). *Journal of Nursing Jocularity's* writer's guidelines. [On-line]. Available: 733314.3032@compuserve.com

Haloob, R. (1984). Oxytocin induced hyponatraemia. *Journal of Obstetrics and Gynecology, 5*(2), 104.

Hanrahan, K. S., Kleiber, C., & Fagan, C. L., (1994). Evaluation of saline for IV locks in children. *Pediatric Nursing, 20*(6), 548–552.

Jacobs, H. B. (1984, September). New York market letter. *Writer's Digest,* 8.

Johnson, S. H. (1992). Getting your research published: Adapting the thesis style. *Nurse Author and Editor, 2*(1), 1–5.

Johnson, S. H. (1993). Nurse author's guide to publishing house editors. *Nurse Author, 3*(3), 3–4, 7.

Lanigan, J., & Miller, J. (1981). Developing Nurse Managers. *Nursing Administration Quarterly, 5*(2), 21–24.

Literary market place. (Annual). New York: R. R. Bowker Co.

Mitchell, M. (1981). The changing role of the nurse in product evaluation. *Nursing Administration Quarterly, 5*(2), 38–42.

Moore-Greenlaw, R. C., & Hurley, M. L. (1994). Nurses are the key to hospital accreditation. *RN, 56*(3), 31–34.

Murray, R. (1993). Home before dark: One nurse's personal experience with diabetic neuropathy. *American Journal of Nursing, 94*(3), 36–42.

News. *American Journal of Nursing* (1993, November), *93*(11), 8.

Pender, N. J. (1993). Research! America: Building public support for research. *Nursing Outlook, 41*(4), 152–153.

Polking, K. (Ed.). (1983). *Writer's encyclopedia.* Cincinnati, OH: Writer's Digest.

Sharber, J. (1994). Oxygen radicals and calcium ion flux: Role in reperfusion injury following AMI. *Dimensions of Critical Care Nursing, 13*, 256–262.

Sheridan, D. R., & Dowdney, D. L. (1984). Survey of nursing and health care journal editors. Unpublished work.

Sheridan, D. R. (1994). It matters which way to you: Facilitating planning. *Nursing Staff Development Insider, 3*(5), 1, 5.

Vivas, M. (1982). Network: Getting into print. *Nursing Outlook, 30*(8), 484.

Walker, D. D., & Madsen, N. (1981). Overview of recent changes in nursing at Stanford. *Nursing Administration Quarterly, 5*(2), 7–14.

Writer's market. (1985). Cincinnati, OH: Writer's Digest.

Wyness, M. A. (1985). Perceptual dysfunction: Nursing assessment and management. *Journal of Neurosurgical Nursing, 17*(2), 105.

Zobel, L. P. (1992). *The travel writer's handbook* (2nd ed.) Cincinnati, OH: Writer's Digest.

8

Write the Manuscript

PREPARATION FOR WRITING

The previous eight chapters have guided you through a rigorous preparation for writing your article. You are now ready to write the first draft.

The most important rule about writing is to plan well, write fast, and edit well later. This principle capsulizes the writing process. "Write in a way that comes easily and naturally to you, using words and phrases that come readily to hand. But do not assume that because you have acted naturally your product is without flaw" (Strunk & White, 1979, p. 70)

Nurse Author & Editor™ is an important source of ongoing information for nursing writers. It is published by Hall Johnson Communications, Inc., 9737 West Ohio Ave., Lakewood, CO 80226. The quarterly publication includes articles that help you develop the slant, organize the ideas, and even avoid writer's block. Several features give the author specific advice on how to write a better manuscript; these features include:

- **Interviews with Editors:** Editors tell what topics are most timely.
- **Writing Style:** Covers a specific writing style problem.
- **Try It!:** A sample of a common writing problem for you to edit.
- **Manuscript Preparation:** Checklists and tips on preparing the manuscript.
- **Rejection Alert:** Examples of problems which cause rejections.
- **Legal/Ethical Aspects:** Getting copyright permissions and what to look for in a publishing contract.
- **Formats:** Describes how to write in a case study, project report, editorial, research, and other formats.

- **Research Style:** How to write methodology, table, and statistical analysis sections.
- **Editorial Board:** How to provide positive-criticism and spot plagiarism problems.
- **Books:** How to develop a book prospectus and negotiate a contract.
- **Consumer Publications:** Writing for the public.
- **Writer's Block:** Practical tips on how you can find time to write.

So far you have been planning. The main ideas in the remainder of the book are about writing fast and editing well. Writing fast offers you the advantages of a free flow exercise in which your style comes through. Writing fast also helps you avoid writer's block.

Material, Supplies, Equipment

Before you begin writing, you will need to gather the materials you need for your most productive writing. You may prefer preparing your first draft by writing in longhand, using word processing, or dictating into a machine and having the draft transcribed. The best method is the one that works best for you and is easily available to you. Handwriting and word processing have the advantage over dictating as they provide text you can look at as you work.

Word Processing

You will have a real advantage if you use word processing. Word processing not only speeds the editing process, it also provides you with continuous clean printouts to edit. Doublespace your writing and leave wide margins (1½ to 2 inches on all sides) for later editing. Writers face a technological challenge: Using hardware and software for writing and editing on computers. Word processing has replaced the typewriter as the writer's primary tool. We have included some information about word processing here because the advantages over using a typewriter are so vast.

Using word processing makes the writing and revising process efficient. In fact, word processing can become an indispensable tool that helps you write, edit, and update your manuscripts quickly. It can also speed up the process of sending query letters and handling all your written communications. Word processing enables you to perform many editing functions such as inserting or deleting a letter, word, paragraph, or page. "Justify," "center," "bold," and "format" commands allow you to change margins, spacing, and general format. In addition, word processing offers you special features such as proportional print and spacing, automatic word counts, readability analyses, grammar checking, automatic indexing, automatic generation of tables of contents, ability to adapt documents easily to the requirements of various styles, ability to recycle old manuscripts into new, ease in editing, and the ability to correct without introducing new errors.

> Most important, the word processor or personal computer has memory. While writing at the terminal, you can conveniently call up anything you may have already stored. You can refer to the raw data in your lab notebooks, to relevant papers or abstracts, and to a reviewer's or an editor's comments you may have received.
> Various spell-checking programs are available and are useful if used *only* to correct typographical errors. Proofreading is still necessary to prevent errors in context ("bow" instead of "bough," etc.); however, proofreading for contextual errors is usually much more efficient if you are not stopping constantly to correct typographical errors. Virtually all spell-checking programs provide for creating custom dictionaries for scientific terms and unusual words. (Day, 1994, p. 87)

Spelling checkers are available with most word processing programs. Spelling checkers quickly review manuscripts and indicate words that do not match its dictionary. Specialized word processing medical dictionaries check medical terms.

Through using word processing, one author found several elements of her writing process changing. Editing on-screen became second nature:

> A second and more exciting change took place. My style of writing responded to the immediacy of the computer. Because changes were instantaneous, I no longer felt attached to my first way of saying something. I allowed myself to change, substitute, rewrite and experiment with words. The result: a freer, looser style, and at the same time, tighter writing. Freezing on 'final drafts' became a thing of the past, because nothing was ever final. I could fine-tune and edit ad infinitum. While I had expected that word processing would smooth a the mechanics of writing, I hadn't anticipated creative benefits—and in fact, I was completely conscious of the change only when forced to use a typewriter. (Rudick, 1984, p. 61)

The *Chicago Guide to Preparing Electronic Manuscripts* (University of Chicago Press, 1987) shows authors how to make the transition from typewriter to computer in style and format. The stylistic guidance is based on *The Chicago Manual of Style* and emphasizes recommendations for using computers to prepare manuscripts. The book also describes the concept of generic coding of the manuscript so that the typesetter's computer can recognize structural elements and special characters to set them in the designated type styles. Another section of the book guides publishers on which manuscripts make good candidates for electronic conversion.

Ursula Springer of Springer Publishing Company in a letter to authors says:

> (Ursula Springer, personal communication, April 1995) As a reflection of Springer's growing technological sophistication, in the Editorial Department all book and journal manuscripts are now submitted to us on disk (with hardcopy printouts). Our journal production is totally computerized. . . . A major topic today is "electronic publishing." This broad term extends from computerized listings of bibliographic information—on OCLC, CD-ROM, or Internet—to the providing of full contents of a book, journal, or other projects in CD-ROM or Internet.

Selecting Good Hardware and Software for Word Processing. Before you attempt to select software, define the specific tasks you need to perform on the computer. Will you be writing articles, books, school papers, or documentation that requires extensive tabulations, graphs, and charts?

Donna Dowdney, who frequently writes articles for publication on the computer industry, recommends that you define your specific needs. Consider the following:

- The equipment's memory capacity. Certain types of writing may benefit from more storage than others. Book authors require more computer memory than article writers.
- The type of operating system. Software dictates the minimum memory and operating system. Writers need to be concerned about the operating system if additional packages will be added in the future for other purposes such as accounting or graphics.
- The reading ease and comprehensibility of the documentation manual.
- The monitor screen. Some people complain of eyestrain from reading computer screens. Select a screen color combination with which you feel comfortable.
- The quality of the printer. Some writers require printers capable of high volume, but are satisfied with low-quality print. Others require high-quality print and low-volume output. Still others need high volume and high quality. Some writers may require two printers, a dot matrix printer for rough drafts and a laser printer for the final product.
- Keyboard comfort. Try various keyboards to determine which is the most comfortable to use.
- Mouse comfort.
- Service. Investigate what is included in the service agreement. What are the costs for repair and replacement of parts and how quickly is repair available?

- Peripherals. Ask about additional equipment you can add such as a modem if you will need to communicate with other writers, publishers, or databases (reference libraries available by telephone computer interconnection).
- Updates. Ask how programs are updated and what the past record of updates has been.
- Telephone "help" numbers. Ask if there is a telephone number you can call if you need help. Then try that number. One user reported calling a service number and reaching a recording that said his call would be returned in two weeks!
- Return exchange privileges. Ask about possible return exchange privileges if you are dissatisfied with the software's performance. Some packages may have a 30-day exchange privilege for upgrading the software.
- Cost of supplies. How much are disks, laser cartridges, ribbons, paper, and other supplies? Are the necessary supplies available locally and from a variety of manufacturers?

Good software must be reliable and do what its manufacturers claim it will do. It must be usable, clear, and convenient to use. It must not produce detrimental results even when operators give unacceptable input or inconsistent commands.

Many editorial offices have now automated and have begun using manuscript-tracking software to handle the details of manuscript submissions and the peer-review process for the thousands of manuscripts that writers submit annually (Dowdney, 1994).

Occupational Hazard in Using Computers. One debilitating occupational hazard for writers results from using computers:

> Endless hours of computer use can take their toll, particularly on wrists and hands. Repetitive keyboarding, awkward posture, and excessive hand force may all lead to discomfort, no matter your age, sex, or even strength. Through a combination of ergonomic factors, however, wrist discomfort can be minimized. These factors include flexible workstation design, good body support, proper posture, and appropriate workstation accessories. In short, by applying the principles of good office ergonomics you can improve working comfort, lessen fatigue, reduce downtime, and increase your productivity. (Purcell, 1994, p. 77)

Dictating Equipment

Because dictating into a machine is the fastest method for producing a draft and because it works well in combination with a guiding outline, Barbara

Brown, editor of *Nursing Administration Quarterly,* prefers dictating to writing. If you have someone transcribe your dictation, request that it be double-spaced to allow room for editing.

In *Make Yourself Clear!* John Morris (1980) claimed that dictating is the most efficient method of producing a first draft because dictating is, on the average, four times faster than longhand. While people speak at speeds of up to 120 words per minute, they cannot write in longhand at more than 30 words per minute.

In addition to the time saved, Morris indicated that using dictating equipment improves quality because "When you are dictating to a machine, you are working much closer to the speed of your mind, and you are not bogged down by the tedious drudgery of longhand" (pp. 169–170).

Morris also claimed that dictating enhances expressing creativity more effectively than any other method because it encourages use of the creative side of your mind. As you talk your ideas into the machine, the creative part of your mind is generating new ideas related to the immediate subject. Before you forget the idea and your way of expressing it, you can dictate it. Your ideas may relate to something you already wrote or plan to write later. In those cases, dictate this creative idea before you forget it with a note to yourself to move it somewhere else in the finished product.

Another advantage of dictating over writing longhand is the decreased likelihood that you will edit during the draft stage. Morris warned against editing at this stage because "the analytical process of editing cannot, for most people, be successfully combined with the creative process of writing" (p. 170). He claimed the longhand writer, unless carefully trained, has great difficulty writing without editing, and thus loses the creative flow of ideas.

Dictating may be practical for nurses who work in administration or academia if they have access to secretarial services for article writing. This usually is not the case; clinical nurses rarely have secretarial services readily available. However, before dismissing this approach, consider calling a secretarial service for a fee schedule. Portable dictating machines and micro cassette recorders are reasonably priced and continue to improve as office technology advances.

READY TO WRITE

Whichever method you use, be sure to gather all your equipment first— sharp #2 pencils, adequate lighting, your favorite type of pen, a good chair, paper, and/or a dictating machine with batteries, if needed. Place your outline nearby. The outline may be either a detailed spoke diagram or a detailed formal outline that you have adjusted based on your editor's feedback to your query letter.

Begin with the first word, and do not allow any interruptions until you have written a draft of the entire article. Avoid the temptation to edit as you write. Editing slows your pace, makes your manuscript choppy, and invites writer's block. If you are missing a piece of information, add a long dash and look up the information later. Do not try to write the perfect opening sentence now, or you will spend unnecessary time on a sentence you will probably rewrite later. Often writers find their opening sentence in line three or four of their first draft.

Carefully use your outline to guide you through the process. Your outline will help you avoid the digressive sidetracking pitfalls of free flow. Follow each numbered ray on your Sun Diagram or major heading on your outline, freely developing related thoughts in more detail as prescribed by subbranches or subheadings. Let your ideas flow in the sequence of the outline, leaving space as needed for missing pieces. Continue until you have written one complete draft of the article, even if it is very rough with numerous gaps. Then put the copy away for a few days.

When you look at it again, it will be with fresh eyes. This is a good time to have your draft typed and to find the information you need to fill in obvious gaps. For example, you may have written "Primary nursing is—." Look up the missing definition. Include citations in your first draft because you will need to use them in your reference list or bibliography later. You may find it convenient to number your "bib" cards and insert just a number into your first draft where you would put a quote so that you do not interrupt your free flow with copying.

ARTICLE INGREDIENTS

Titles

The basic ingredients of your article include the title, opening paragraph, substance of the manuscript, and conclusion. Since the title is the first part of your article that the reader notices, the title must have impact on the reader. "A title is more than a label for a story: it is a theme. It not only tells the editor what you're trying to say, but also keeps you on the track yourself" (McKinney, 1983, p. 31).

Gordon Wells (1983) listed several title categories: labels, questions, quotations, exclamatory statements, and puns. The following are examples of each type of title.

Label

- "Readership Survey Report" (McCoy, 1994)
- "Developing a Paper Presentation" (Pierce & Gregg, 1994)
- "Electronic Scholarly Publishing and The World Wide Web" (Treloar, 1996)

Question

- "What Is a Book Review?" (Dreher, 1983)
- "Ethics: Authorship in Biomedical Publication: 'How many people can wield one pen?'" (McLellan, 1995)
- "Where Does Scholarly Electronic Publishing Get You?" (Butler, 1995)
- "Is My Book Idea Sellable? Writing the Book Proposal" (McCormick, 1992)

Quotation/Saying

- "Publish or Perish: How to Accomplish the Former and Avoid the Latter" (Overfield, 1981)
- "Perishing While Publishing: As the Editor Sees It" (Lewis, 1980b)

Exclamatory Statement

- "You Can Write!" (Robinson, 1982)

Pun

- "A Peerless Publication" (Lewis, 1980a)
- "Teching It Easy" (Rudick, 1984)
- "Double Time"—an article about collaboration (Watson-Rouslin & Peck, 1985)

A title with a pun is generally not a good choice for a professional article because indexers use the title to determine the appropriate category in which to index the article. Look at the working title you selected earlier and consider the possibilities above to determine if you want to refine the title at this point. After you select a working title, you are ready to plan the lead sentence and paragraph.

Topic Sentences

Begin your manuscript by creating a topic sentence for your first paragraph. The topic sentence states the subject and controlling idea of the paragraph. Every other sentence in the paragraph develops and supports the controlling idea about which you wrote the topic sentence. Look at your Sun Diagram for potential topic sentences.

Although your topic sentence will usually be the first sentence in each paragraph, you can place it in other positions, depending on the emphasis you want to achieve. Typical positions for topic sentences are at the beginning, middle, and end of paragraphs. Summarize each paragraphs's controlling idea through its topic sentences. Effective topic sentences give clues about your paragraph's organization.

In the previous chapter, you developed a lead sentence to use in your query letter. Now you may be able to use that lead sentence as your topic sentence in your first paragraph.

> The lead must capture the reader immediately and force him to keep reading. It must cajole him with freshness or novelty or paradox, or with humor, or with surprise, or with an unusual idea, or an interesting fact, or a question. Anything will do as long as it nudges his curiosity and tugs at his sleeve . . . the lead must provide a few hard details that tell the reader why the piece was written and why he ought to read it. But don't dwell on the reason. Coax the reader a little more; keep him inquisitive. . . . Continue to build. Every paragraph should amplify the one that preceded it. (Zinsser, 1980, p. 60)

Your lead sentence is vital because if it does not lead the reader to continue to the second and third sentences, you article will not be read. In the same way, the lead paragraph should grab the reader's attention and lead the reader through the rest of your article.

> The lead paragraph should establish the what, where, when, how, why, and who for the reader. If the subject is of interest to him, he will read on. Or, if the lead is clever, he will proceed further before he makes his decision to continue. (Robinson & Notter, 1982, p. 15)

Developing Paragraphs

After you write your lead sentence and paragraph, you will use the framework you selected earlier to build the remainder of the article. To write effective paragraphs, use examples and details to back up the topic sentence. You have several choices in how to develop your paragraphs. You could use narrative, explanation, description, sequence/chronology, comparison/contrast, cause/effect, pro/con, or definition. You may select from several patterns for developing each paragraph. A few of the more commonly used patterns include definition, analysis, generalization, and classification.

Paragraphs are groups of sentences that both develop and support one central idea. The paragraph's primary purpose is to develop the idea you state in your topic sentence. Good paragraphs are unified, coherent, and developed appropriately.

Think of each paragraph as a brick in a building. Each brick builds on those below and adjacent to it. Each brick contributes to the wall's strength and beauty. Just as a fine mason would not insert unnecessary bricks into a wall, so in your writing resist any temptation to add ideas and words to your paragraphs that do not contribute to making your paragraph strong.

Good paragraphs are ones that are adequately developed, unified, and coherent. Each paragraph reveals its unity because it relates to and contributes to the topic sentence. Readers recognize coherence in paragraphs because they can easily see how one idea relates to the next. By using related terms that show how the paragraph focuses on one idea, you build coherence.

Parallel grammatical structure also emphasizes a paragraph's coherence. For example, Welches, in "The Practicing Nurse as Nurse Researcher" (1983), opened her article with a paragraph using parallel structure:

> Nursing research is one of the most powerful instruments available to the practicing nurse today. When integrated as a part of nursing practice, nursing research will lead to more scientifically based practice, to improvement of patient care, and to containment of the costs of that care. (p. 17)

Length of Paragraphs

How long should your paragraphs be? "A good rule of thumb is that a paragraph should be just long enough to deal adequately with the subject of its topic sentence. A new paragraph should begin wherever the subject changes significantly" (Brusaw, Alred, & Oliu, 1993, p. 494). Vary your paragraph length to help keep the reader's interest and attention. Generally, scholarly articles have longer and more complex paragraphs than articles intended for lighter reading.

Checklist for Effective Paragraphs

- Does each paragraph express one thought?
- Does each sentence contribute to developing the topic sentence?

- Does each paragraph contribute to the article as a whole?
- Does each paragraph seem to be in its logical place?
- Do the length and pattern of the sentences within each paragraph vary?
- Does each paragraph have a topic sentence?

RESPONSIBLE WRITING

Citations and Paraphrasing

Use citations liberally to ensure that you are not taking credit for someone else's work. A common error writers make is to misuse paraphrasing. Some writers incorrectly assume that if they change one or two words in a passage they are paraphrasing. Be sure to credit paraphrased ideas and words to their original writers.

Plagiarism, Libel, and Invasion of Privacy

Plagiarism involves using or closely imitating someone else's writing without obtaining their permission, acknowledging, or compensating them and representing it as your own. To avoid plagiarism, give credit to your sources. Obtain written permission from copyright owners to use their copyrighted material in your manuscript.

Christine Chapman (1980) wrote, "To include any of anyone else's work or ideas in an article without making reference to their source is plagiarism because it conveys the impression that the phrase and/or the idea belongs to the writer of the article. This constitutes a theft of words or ideas, things which are the properly of another" (p. 1160).

The "Letters to the Editor" column in the May 1982 issue of *Nursing Outlook* presented nurses' concerns on literary piracy. Some nurses were concerned about whether to grant permission to tape lectures, speeches, or workshops when the material was original and not yet published. Other issues raised were about verbatim copying of questions and using someone else's original doctoral work without acknowledgment of that person's contributions to the field. All these areas involve the question of whether attribution or citation is required. Our view is whenever in doubt, include a citation.

In an editorial in the May 1980 issue of *AORN*, Elinor S. Schrader wrote, "At best, plagiarism is the result of ignorance; at worst, it is dishonesty or the attempt to represent ideas, thoughts, and words of others as one's own. It is intellectual theft" (p. 981).

Libel is written or published defamation or injury to someone's name or reputation. Although statements are not libelous if they are true, proving their truth may be quite difficult. The following are some examples of libel.

Suppose you were writing an article on "How Available Are Doctors at Night?" In your article, you state, without thorough investigation, that several patients have died in your hospital because physicians were not available at night. Somewhere in your article the hospital is named or is easily identified; the physicians could be recognized from your description of facts. A nursing journal would probably never publish this article unless it were edited for this problem. However, if it were published, the author and the journal would have committed libel. Libel may result in expensive damage suits and a loss of your professional reputation.

Other potential sources of libel might stem from unfounded and undocumented criticisms of hospitals, health agencies, or health care providers. Validate all facts, especially any comments that could negatively affect someone's reputation.

Unfounded criticism of drug or medical supply companies could also lead to court action. Other consequences might be published retractions or withdrawal of your article for publication. If your criticisms are in direct conflict with a publication's advertisers, your article may not be considered for publication.

Also be careful to avoid invasion of privacy. This involves using information about someone's private life for your profit or gain. Be sure to obtain written permission to use photographs of patients and colleagues. You also need permission to identify a patient by name unless the circumstances have been changed sufficiently to prevent identification (e.g., age, date of incident, sex, etc.).

FILLING IN GAPS

Do not attempt to write a second draft until you have filled in the gaps in your first draft. Then watch for other more subtle gaps such as lack of transitions between sections as you read your manuscript. Check if you need to substantiate or clarify a thought with a definition or question.

In addition, before you write a second draft, be sure to number your pages and indicate what number draft this is. For example, label your first page DIp1 (for Draft I page 1). You may want to change the color of paper or pen for each draft.

Experienced nurse authors in our survey were asked how many drafts they write. The average number of drafts was three, although the numbers varied between 1 and 10 drafts. One person said, "I write as many drafts as needed" (Sheridan & Dowdney, 1984).

Your second draft may involve filling in gaps, reordering sentences, smoothing out or clarifying thoughts, adding examples and citations, or identifying rough transitions between thoughts. Edit by using a red pen (or some different color from draft #1) and by writing between the lines or in the margins. If you have long insertions, write "Insert A here" on the draft and begin sequential pages of lettered inserts. After you fill in the gaps, you are ready to revise your manuscript. The steps for revision are covered in the next chapter.

Count the Words

Count the words in your manuscript. It is important to find out whether you are only half finished, or if you have written twice as much as you need! You can make a quick estimate by counting the number of words in ten lines and then determining the average number of words per line. Then count the lines on an average page and multiply by the average word number. Some word processing programs automatically indicate how many words are in your manuscript. Generally, nursing and health care articles are about 2,000 words in length, but this can vary greatly from journal to journal and even within one journal. Do not worry if your manuscript is too long. Good editing will reduce most free flow drafts by a third or more. Clarity and conciseness are essential to a well-written manuscript.

EXERCISES

1. Gather your equipment and supplies for writing.
2. Begin writing your manuscript.

REFERENCES

Brusaw, C. T., Alred, G. J., & Oliu, W. E. (1993). *Handbook of technical writing.* New York: St. Martin's.

Butler, H. (1995). Where does scholarly electronic publishing get you? *Journal of Scholarly Publishing, 26,* 174.

Chapman, C. (1980). Plagiarism—a form of stealing. *Nursing Times, 76*(27), 1160.

Day, R. A. (1994). *How to write and publish a scientific paper.* Phoenix, Oryx Press.

Dowdney, D. L. (1994). Editorial tracking software. *CBE Views, 17*(5), 81.

Dreher, M. C. (1983). What is a book review? *Nursing Outlook, 31*(1), 64.

Letters to the editor. (1982, May). *Nursing Outlook, 30,* 278–279.

Lewis, E. P. (1980a). A peerless publication. *Nursing Outlook, 28*(4), 225–226.

Lewis, E. P. (1980b, November 28). Perishing while publishing: As the editor sees it. *Nursing Outlook, 28*(11), 689–690.

McCormick, M. (1992). Is my book idea sellable? Writing the book proposal. *Nurse Author, 2*(3), 7–9.

McCoy, K. (1994). Readership survey report. *Insight, 19*(2), 28–29.

McKinney, D. (1983, September). How to make your articles sparkle. *Writer's Digest,* 31.

McLellan, M. F. (1995). Ethics: Authorship in biomedical publication: "How many people can wield one pen?" *AMWA Journal, 10*(1), 11.

Morris, J. O. (1980). *Make yourself clear* (pp. 169–170). New York: McGraw-Hill.

Overfield, T. (1981). Publish or perish: How to accomplish the former and avoid the latter. *Western Journal of Nursing Research, 3*(4), 417–420.

Pierce, L. L., & Gregg, M. M. (1994). Developing a paper presentation. *Rehabilitation Nursing, 19*(3), 151–155.

Purcell, T. J. (1994). Ergonomics and the writer. *AMWA Journal, 9*(2), 77.

Robinson, A. M. (1982). You can write! *Imprint, 29*(5), 48.

Robinson, A. M., & Notter, L. E. (1982). *Clinical writing for health professionals.* Bowie, MD: Robert J. Brady Co.

Rudick, M. (1984, May). Teching it easy. *Writer's Digest,* 61.

Schrader, E. S. (1980, May). Perils and pitfalls of plagiarism and how to avoid them. *AORN Journal, 31,* 981–982.

Sheridan, D. R., & Dowdney, D. L. (1984). Survey of selected nurse authors. Unpublished work.

Strunk, W., Jr., & White, E. B. (1979). *The elements of style.* New York: Macmillan.

Treloar, A. (1996). Electronic scholarly publishing and the World Wide Web. *Journal of Scholarly Publishing, 27,* 135.

University of Chicago Press. (1987). *Chicago guide to preparing electronic manuscripts.* Chicago: Author.

Watson-Rouslin, V., & Peck, J. M. (1985, March). Double time. *Writer's Digest,* 32.

Welches, L. J. (1983). The practicing nurse as nurse researcher. *The Journal of Burn Care and Rehabilitation, 4*(1), 17–18.

Wells, G. (1983). *The craft of writing articles.* London: Allison & Busby.

Writer's guidelines. (1995). *Journal of Nursing Jocularity.*

Zinsser, W. (1980). *On writing well.* New York: Harper & Row.

9

Revise the Manuscript

By going through your manuscript step by step looking for grammatical and stylistic errors, you will find your own pitfalls—the writing errors you are most likely to commit. Thus, each time you edit you will become faster and better. Remember, write fast for style and flow of ideas; then edit well.

In our survey of nursing journal editors, we asked, "What are the most common grammatical errors present in submitted manuscripts?" In addition to spelling, capitalization, punctuation, and typographical errors, editors identified the following areas:

- Noun–verb agreement; plural verbs and singular nouns.
- Convoluted, unwieldy, complicated sentence structure.
- Pretentious prose with overuse of jargon.
- Run-on sentences.
- Wordiness and redundancy.
- Too much passive voice.
- Modifiers removed from the word being modified.
- Awkward wording.
- Shifting from singular to plural.
- Shifting from first person to third person.
- Mixing verb tenses.
- Improper use of scientific nomenclature.
- Misuse of prepositions.
- Misuse of nouns as verbs.
- Dangling participles.
- Misuse of pronouns such as "this" and "which."
- Lack of flow of thought and transitions.

In this chapter we show you how to revise your manuscript to increase clarity and improve style as well as how to recognize unnecessary verbiage and redundancies. The chapter shows you how to add variety and emphasis to your sentences and how to use transitions, headings, and parallel sentence structures effectively. This chapter helps you identify problems with sexist, stereotypical, and dehumanizing words. It also shows you how to transform vague words into specific, concrete terms. A revision checklist and nine principles for improving your writing conclude the chapter.

Now that you have written your first draft, you are ready to begin revising to see if your manuscript contains any of the above common grammatical problems. After we explain each revision area, we use an asterisk to indicate that a brief exercise follows. When you see the asterisk, examine your manuscript for the problem described in that section.

Begin revising by reading the draft aloud to discover weak spots and areas that need additional work. Look for thoughts that are inaccurate, incomplete, unclear, or wordy. Although it is beyond the scope of this book to deal in depth with grammatical, punctuation, and spelling problems, we have included a brief overview of basic grammatical and writing concepts to help you avoid common writing pitfalls and prepare a publishable manuscript.

BASIC GRAMMATICAL TERMS

Grammatical terms define the basic structure of a language and how it works. As a writer, you will need to communicate precisely, directly, and clearly by using your basic tool—language. Understanding the basic grammatical concepts is essential for identifying problem areas. Knowledge of basic grammatical concepts will guide you in avoiding and/or correcting your writing problems. Gary Provost said:

> There are two large groups of people who are wrong about grammar and, generally speaking, neither group produces good writers. One group comprises people who think they can ignore the rules of grammar altogether and still write successfully by scribbling any combination of words that occurs to them, while announcing to the world that ignorance or laziness is really artistic freedom. The people in the other group are those who discuss grammar as if it were some sort of religion that must be rigidly followed even if clarity, wit, style and poetry must be sacrificed. They would rather be right than write well. Both groups make the same mistake. They view grammar as a master when they should look upon it as a servant. (Provost, 1984, p. 37)

Provost went on to say:

> To succeed as a writer, you must know, respect and obey the rules of grammar in your writing. . . . Good writing and good grammar are not twins, but they are usually found in the same places. The rules of grammar exist to help you write well, not to sabotage your work, and you cannot write well without them. The rules of grammar organize the language just as the rules of arithmetic organize the world of numbers. (Provost, 1984, p. 37)

The following is a brief review of a few common parts of speech: nouns, pronouns, verbs, adjectives, and adverbs. Each time we present a part of speech, we identify its particular features that cause problems for writers and give opportunities for you to examine your manuscript for possible problems in these areas.

Identifying parts of speech can be a confusing process because the same word can work as different parts of speech, depending on the sentence in which it appears. For example, most people think of "nurse" only as a noun: "The student is a *nurse*." However, "nurse" can also be used as a verb: "The woman *will nurse* her elderly parents back to health."

"Drug" can also be used as various parts of speech: "The *drugs* were locked in the cabinet" (noun). "The *drugged* derelict slept on the sidewalk" (adjective). "The experiment involved *drugging* the subject" (gerund—verb form used as a noun).

Because words can be used in various contexts as different parts of speech, and because the language is constantly changing, the following simple definitions and examples will help you identify a word's part of speech in the context of specific sentences.

Nouns

You can tell if a word is a noun by asking questions. If the answer is "yes" to the following questions, the word probably is a noun.

- Does a "noun determiner" precede the word? Noun determiners include the following: the, a, an, my, your, our, their, this, these, that, those, his, her, its, one . . . ninety-nine, many, more, several, both, all, some, no, every, a few, other, enough
- Does the word have any of the following endings?: -'s, -es, -age, -ance, -ee, -ment, -ce, -cy, -ity, -ness, -ster, -cy, -er, -ian, -ism, -ist, -ship, -ster, or -er.
- Does the word precede a verb?
- Does the word name a person, place, object, concept, or activity? Examples are Susan, Chicago, hospital, health, and writing.

- Does the word function as a noun in the sentence? If the word functions as a subject (the naming part of the sentence) or object (something that receives the action of the verb), it is a noun.

One problem writers frequently have with nouns is using too many nouns together so that they create "noun chains." In *Nursing Outlook,* Ellen Goldensohn (1982, p. 541) described the appearance of noun chains in writing: "At first, nouns may appear in seemingly innocuous pairs (health behaviors, communication facilitation, intimacy skills). Soon afterward, clusters appear (health maintenance techniques, support system network)."

Then Goldensohn described indiscriminate noun chains taking over entire sentences as in "Communication facilitation skills development intervention." She concluded, "The disease has reached an acute stage and should be treated aggressively."

You can convert some noun chains into other parts of speech. For example, you could change "health maintenance techniques" to "techniques for maintaining health."

Search your manuscript for noun chains. If you find any, try various ways of rephrasing the noun chains by converting them into other parts of speech.

Pronouns

Pronouns take the place of nouns and refer to the same person or object as a nearby noun. Examples of pronouns include: I, we, you, he, she, it, they, who, me, my, mine, us, our, ours, him, his, her, hers, it, its, them, their, theirs, who, whom, whose, anyone, anybody, anything, each, either, everybody, everyone, everything, neither, nobody, nothing, one, somebody, someone, and something.

A writer's primary problem with pronouns is the ambiguity that results when readers cannot easily discover the exact word to which the pronoun refers. Frequently ambiguity results from beginning a new sentence or paragraph with a pronoun such as "this," "it," or "that." Such sentence beginnings force readers to return to the previous sentence or paragraph to discover the word to which the pronoun refers.

Other examples of confusing pronoun references appear in the following sentences:

- "The primary nurse was giving medication to the patient, and she looked distressed." In this sentence the reader can not tell who "she" is.
- "One of the patients informed the nurse that she didn't understand the procedure." Who did not understand the procedure, the nurse or the patient?

- "Cost containment is essential for health care. It is economically essential in a nation that values a high quality of life." What does "it" refer to, "cost containment" or "health care"?

Sometimes sentences with ambiguous pronoun references result in unplanned humor, for example, "If you have headaches, the nurse will examine your eyes and help you eliminate them." To remove the ambiguity in this sentence, write, "If you have headaches, the nurse will examine your eyes. Examining your eyes may help find the cause so we can eliminate your headaches." Another example is "We don't tear your linen with machinery. We do it carefully by hand." To remove the ambiguity in this sentence, say, "We don't tear your linen by using machinery. Instead, we wash your linen by hand."

Another problem with pronouns involves the relative pronouns "which" and "that." These pronouns relate a subordinate clause to its main clause. Use "which" for nonrestrictive clauses and "that" for restrictive ones. In "The bacteria that caused the disease has not been determined," the clause "that caused the disease" is restrictive. The writer is defining the particular bacteria involved; the clause cannot be omitted without changing the meaning of the sentence. "Which" clauses are nonrestrictive, which means they can be dropped without changing the basic meaning of the sentence. These clauses are parenthetical rather than central to the meaning of the sentence, and are set off with commas, for example, "The thermometer, which was digital, was more accurate."

Examine every pronoun in your manuscript to make certain each one is clear in its reference. Give particular attention to any paragraphs beginning with this, that, or it.

Verbs

Verbs name actions (laugh, drive, job) or states of being (am, is, was, were, being, been). Other words often used as verbs or helping verbs include: can, could, must, may, might, shall, should, will, would, do, does, did, get, gets, got, have, had, and has. Sometimes "en-" or "em-" appears before nouns to transform them into verbs (embitter or enlighten).

Voice.   Verbs have two voices: active and passive. Voice shows whether the subject is acting (active) or being acted upon (passive). Frequently writers overuse passive voice, which can make sentences awkward and dull. Sentences often are more effective when they are in active voice because the sentence tells who does what.

The active voice places the responsibility for the design of the study, the protocol, the methods, and the conclusions squarely where it belongs—on the shoulders of the investigators and ultimately the author or authors. . . . It is not "more scientific" and "objective" to use the passive voice; it is only more imprecise—and cowardly. However, circumstances sometimes necessitate use of the passive voice to avoid absurdities or convoluted phraseology. Here, as everywhere and always, good sense and judgment—hallmarks of the good editor—will prevail and will suggest the choice. If it is not really important to know which specific unit did the laboratory studies, for example, the passive voice is appropriate. . . Using the active voice may even make a specific paper or book more lively as well as informative. It is possible to write factually *and* interestingly. The pity is that it is so seldom done, sometimes because of an unwarranted fear that the reader will think less of the author, her or his scientific objectivity, or the work if the manuscript is interesting. (Schwager, 1991, pp. 41–42)

- PASSIVE: "Watching the remarkable postoperative recovery was enjoyed by the clinic staff."
- ACTIVE: "The clinic staff enjoyed watching the remarkable postoperative recovery."
- PASSIVE: "The guidelines to improve the quality of charting were approved by the entire staff."
- ACTIVE: "The entire staff approved the guidelines to improve the practice of charting."

In active voice, the subject performs the action. Active voice adds interest, sparkle, and punch to writing. It shortens sentences and increases their impact.

The following guidelines will help you decide whether active or passive voice is most appropriate to use in your sentences:

- Use active voice if the doer is more important than the recipient. ("The nurse inoculated the patient against cholera.")
- Use passive voice if the recipient of the action is more important than the doer of the action. ("The patient had been inoculated against cholera.")
- Use passive voice if the doer of the action is unknown or unimportant. ("The operation had been completed.")
- Use passive voice to slow the reader and de-emphasize who is responsible. ("The medication had been misplaced.")
- Use passive voice to be tactful and avoid placing blame. ("The charts had been removed from the nursing station and were found in the lounge.")

Look for passive voice in your manuscript. Wherever it is appropriate, trans-form passive to active voice.

Smothered Verbs and Pretentious Prose.   One common mistake writers make is smothering strong verbs by changing them into nouns. In smoth-ering the verbs, writers create pretentious prose that may sound impres-sive but is actually weak, for example, "Authorization for the absence was given by the nurse supervisor." You could improve this sentence by trans-forming the noun "authorization" into its verb form, "authorize." Write, "The nurse supervisor authorized the absence."

If you tend to use words ending in "-ion," "-tion," "iation," "-ment," or "-ance," remove these endings and transform the nouns into strong work-ing verbs. Examples of nouns that could be transformed into verbs include: authorization, documentation, negotiation, illustration, concession, imple-mentation, quotation, advancement, employment, significance, and com-pliance.

Leah L. Curtin, editor of *Nursing Management,* wrote:

> Occasionally, I suspect that people resort to pretentious prose when they really don't have anything important to say; when they don't know how to say what they want to say; when they want what they have to say to sound more important than it is; or when they have to say something controversial, unpopular or unpleasant and they haven't the courage to say it in plain Eng-lish. (1981, p. 7)

She pointed out that the purpose of speaking or writing is to communicate, not to confuse, and that many manuscripts are rejected because they are too difficult to understand. She then asked readers to consider the following exam-ple: "The nurse managers responded to a burgeoning census and escalating acuity by extrapolating data that enabled the finalization and implementation of a program which incorporated a conceptually meaningful approach to all parameters of holistic care which, in turn, impacted positively on patients." Curtin asked, "What does this mean?" She pointed out that the number, com-plexity and misuse of the words set up impossible obstacles for the reader.

She continued:

> Why can't we just use something, why do we have to utilize it? What's wrong with thinking instead of conceptualizing? Why don't we do things anymore, rather than operationalize them? Do long words sound more impressive than their smaller (and usually more accurate) counterparts? There may be times when the use of long words is appropriate. However, substituting an impres-sive sounding, long word is intolerable when the word isn't used correctly. (Curtin, 1981, p. 7)

In her editorial "Pretentious Prose" in *Nursing Outlook,* Edith P. Lewis observed, "We no longer have factors or dimensions, we have parameters. We don't generalize, we extrapolate. Things don't fit well together, they interface. And we don't even work in a hospital any more, but in a hospital setting" (Lewis, 1974, p. 431).

Although sometimes "conceptualized," "extrapolate," or "parameter" is the appropriate word, often writers substitute the more impressive word for the smaller one without considering the exact meaning of either one. In doing this the words become devalued and their specific meaning is blurred.

In *Nursing Mirror,* George Castledine (1982) wrote about the increasing use of jargon by nurses:

> Take for example the use of the term "nursing process" or some of the words used to describe nursing actions. . . . A certain amount of nursing jargon is inevitable and probably necessary, but it is when it becomes pretentious and unnecessarily complex or obscure that it no longer serves a useful purpose. (Castledine, 1982, p. 31)

The unnecessary creation of new words from old by adding "-ize," "-wise," and "-ate" to make words such as "operationalize," "finalize," "maximize," "prioritize," "optimize," "potentialize," "media-wise," and "effectuate" further contributes to pretentious prose.

Check your manuscript for any examples of smothered verbs or pretentious prose. Transform the smothered verbs into strong working verbs. Delete the pretentious prose.

Adjectives

Adjectives modify or describe nouns or pronouns and answer the following questions: "What kind?" (Poor, excellent, mediocre.) "How many?" (Three, fifty.) "Which one?" (The latest, the fastest.)

One problem writers have with adjectives is using a modifier for a compound term. For example, "kidney function examination" could refer to a function test for kidneys or an examination applied to kidney function. Another compound term is "toxic shock syndrome." Does this refer to a syndrome of toxic shock or a shock syndrome? A solution to this problem could be to use hyphens to indicate linkage, such as in "kidney-function examination."

Another modifier problem is ambiguity. Keep modifiers close to the words they modify. Otherwise misinterpretation or undesired humor can result. For example, "Pass the surgeon across the sterile field the forceps."

This sentence is unclear as to whether to pass the forceps or the surgeon and results in unplanned humor. To make the sentence clearer, write, "Pass the forceps across the field to the surgeon."

Another example of a modifier creating ambiguity is "About to overflow, the nurse emptied the thoracic drainage." What was about to overflow, the nurse or the drainage? The corrected sentence reads: "The nurse emptied the thoracic drainage that was about to overflow."

Review your manuscript for misplaced and ambiguous modifiers.

Verbals

Verbals are derived from verbs but do not function as verbs in sentences. Categories of verbals include infinitives ("to" with a verb—" to inoculate"); present participles ("-ing" form of a verb used as a verb or modifier—"distressing"); and past participles ("-ed" form in some verbs). In other words, verbals are verb forms that are not used as verbs within sentences; they function as other parts of speech.

One type of verbal, the participle, causes particular difficulty for writers. Sometimes people refer to the problem as "dangling participles." The most common problem writers have with dangling modifiers is illustrated in the following sentence: "Failing to locate the problem, the plan for discharge was altered." Who or what was failing to locate the problem? Replace the words following the introductory words and comma with a subject or rephrase the sentence: "Failing to locate the problem, the physician altered the discharge."

Another example of a dangling participle is, "Having demonstrated the procedure, expectations of students were raised." To improve this sentence, tell who demonstrated the procedure. "After the preceptor demonstrated the procedure, she raised her expectations of students."

Review your manuscript for dangling participles and rewrite any confusing sentences.

Adverbs

Adverbs modify or describe verbs, adjectives, or other adverbs. They answer the following questions: When? (now); Where? (here); In what manner? (slowly); To what extent? (completely). Overuse of adverbs can weaken your writing. Particularly avoid "very," "really," and "little." Most adverbs are unnecessary because they lengthen sentences and duplicate the meaning of verbs. Take the following sentence, "The ambulance siren blared loudly." "Blared" means "loudly." In "The patient clenched his fist tightly," "clench" means to hold tightly.

Delete the words "very," "little," and "really" from your manuscript. Then look for any other adverbs you used that duplicate a verb.

Prepositional Phrases

A phrase is a group of words not containing a verb and its subject. A preposition shows the relationship of a noun or a pronoun to other words in a sentence. Commonly used prepositions include: about, above, across, after, against, along, amid, among, around, at, before, behind, below, beneath, beside, besides, between, beyond, but (meaning "except"), by, concerning, down, during, except, for, from, in, into, like, of, off, on, over, past, since, through, throughout, to, toward, under, underneath, until, unto, up, upon, with, within, and without. Groups of words can work together as prepositions such as "in the event that" or "in spite of."

A prepositional phrase begins with a preposition and ends with a noun or pronoun, for example: to the nurse; after the exam; in the hospital; during the operation. The noun or pronoun that ends the prepositional phrase is the object of the preposition.

Too many prepositional phrases in sentences contribute to wordiness. Count the prepositional phrases in the following paragraph: "The use of a theoretical framework about crisis intervention in the presentation of the class to teach about emergency nursing of the trauma patient is useful throughout the theory segment of the teaching, but not as much during the teaching section concerning care of this type of patient in the practical sense." This paragraph uses 13 prepositional phrases. Did you find all of them?

The following revision decreases the number of prepositional phrases from 13 to 2: "A crisis intervention framework is useful in teaching the theoretical, not the practical, segment of nursing the trauma patient."

Search your manuscript for groups of prepositional phrases. Eliminate unnecessary ones. By removing unnecessary prepositional phrases, you will also make your writing more concise.

WORDINESS AND REDUNDANCY

Strunk and White (1979, p. *xiv*) wrote:

> Vigorous writing is concise. A sentence should contain no unnecessary words, a paragraph no unnecessary sentences, for the same reason that a drawing should have no unnecessary lines and a machine no unnecessary parts. This requires not that the writer make all his sentences short, or that he avoid all detail and treat his subjects only in outline, but that every word tell.

Sometimes a pair of words does the work of one word; such redundancy violates conciseness. Redundant word combinations include "originally began," "refer back," "over with," "cooperate together," and "exactly identical."

Eliminate unnecessary prepositional phrases and redundancies. Concise replacements are included in Table 9.1.

William Zinsser, in *On Writing Well*, wrote:

> Clutter is the disease of American writing. We are a society strangling in unnecessary words, circular constructions, pompous frills, and meaningless jargon. . . . The secret of good writing is to strip every sentence to its cleanest components. Every word that serves no function, every long word that could be a short word, every adverb which carries the same meaning that is already in the verb, every passive construction that leaves the reader unsure of who is doing what—these are the thousand and one adulterants that weaken the strength of a sentence. And they usually occur, ironically, in proportion to education and rank. (Zinsser, 1980, pp. 7–8)

Review your manuscript for wordiness and redundancies. Eliminate unnecessary words. Prune brutally without losing the thought.

ENGLISH SENTENCE PATTERNS

If you can recognize the following English sentence patterns in your writing, you will be able to vary them to avoid monotonous writing. The five patterns are:

1. *Subject-Verb:* "Nurses plan." In this pattern, the subject precedes the verb. The subject of a sentence must agree in number with the verb. That is, if the subject is singular, the verb also must be singular: "The patient is conscious" (singular subject and verb). "The patients are conscious" (plural subject and verb).

A common pitfall in agreement occurs when the subject and verb are separated by a prepositional phrase, for example, "He is one of those nurses who believe in his own ability." This should read: "He is one of those nurses who *believes* in his own ability." When you temporarily remove a prepositional phrase, you are able to see the subject and verb that should agree.

2. *Subject-Verb-Object:* "Nurses plan care." The object, *care* in this sentence, receives the verb's action. Direct objects are nouns or pronouns.

3. *Subject-Verb-Indirect Object-Direct Object:* "The nurse gave the patient the treatment." The direct object answers the question "What?" What did

Table 9.1. Eliminating Wordiness

Wordy	Concise
Square in shape	square
Green in color	green
Many in number	many
An order of magnitude greater than	greater than
In my opinion, I think	I think
Thirty-year period of time	thirty years
Duration of time	duration
Consensus of opinion	consensus
In a hasty mannner	hastily
In excess of	more than
For the purposes of	to or so
In the event that	if
The question as to whether	whether
In an effort to	to
For the length of time that	while
Pertains to the problem of	concerns
To be of great benefit	beneficial
Could be felt by the hand	felt
Reliable in character	reliable
Tasted sour to the tongue	sour
Third time in my life	third time
As of this date	today
In this day and age	today
At the present time	now
For the reason that	because
In view of	because
Due to the fact that	because
In the amount of	for
In the event of	if
A majority of	most
A number of	several
Accounted for by the fact that	because
Under the current circumstances	as things are
Are of the same opinion	agree
At this point in time	now
As a consequence of	because
By means of	by
On account of	because
Is of the opinion that	believed
At a period of time when	when
With a view to	to
With the result that	so

the nurse give? The treatment. "Treatment" is the direct object of the verb "gave." Indirect objects answer the questions "To whom?" or "For whom?" Thus, in the sentence above, "the patient" is the indirect object of the verb. "To whom did the nurse give the treatment?" "The patient."

4. *Subject-Verb-Predicate Noun:* "The nurse is the patient's advocate." Predicate nouns follow a special kind of verb called a "linking verb" (am, is, be, are, was, were, been, seem, appear, become, and remain). Predicate nouns are interchangeable with the subject. For example, you could either say "The nurse is the patient's advocate" or "The patient's advocate is the nurse." One of these nouns functions as the subject, the other as the predicate noun.

5. *Subject-Verb-Predicate Adjective:* "The instruction is skilled." The predicate adjective modifies or describes the subject and follows the linking verb "is."

Find an example of each of the five sentence types in your writing. Have you used all five? If not, try incorporating each sentence type in order to increase variety in your writing.

COMPLEXITY OF SENTENCES

In addition to examining sentences for sentence patterns (order of the parts of speech), sentences can be analyzed in terms of complexity. The four major levels of complexity in sentences are categorized as simple, complex, compound, and compound-complex. After you analyze your writing for sentence patterns, look at complexity to assure variety in this aspect of your writing.

The key to analyzing complexity is clauses. There are two primary kinds of clauses: independent and dependent. Independent clauses, which can stand alone as sentences, have a subject and verb and express a complete thought. Although dependent clauses have subjects and verbs, they do not express a complete thought and depend on another part of the sentence for meaning.

Simple Sentences

A simple sentence has one independent clause with no dependent clauses attached. However, it may have modifying phrases. "The patient went to the operating room" is an example of a simple sentence. Use a simple sentence when you want to make unqualified observations. Use a simple sentence to emphasize ideas, but beware of overusing simple sentences because your writing will sound choppy, simplistic, or condescending.

When two simple sentences have the same subject, combine them by dropping the subject of the second sentence and adding connecting words. For example, if you have two simple sentences such as "The charge nurse wrote the assignments. The charge nurse posted the assignments," combine them: "The charge nurse wrote and posted the assignments."

Complex Sentences

A complex sentence has one independent clause and one or more dependent clauses that express subordinate ideas, for example, "Although anorexia nervosa is usually found in young women, it is occasionally found in young men."

Subordination involves using dependent clauses, phrases, or single words to express ideas that are not significant enough to be expressed in an independent clause. For example: "Abraham Maslow constructed a theory. His theory was about motivation. He said that people have unmet needs. Unmet needs are motivators." This sounds simplistic and choppy. Change it to "Abraham Maslow, in his theory of motivation, said people's unmet needs are motivators."

Here is an example of lack of subordination: "The wound began to drain purulent material. The patient's temperature spiked to 103.2 degrees Fahrenheit." Subordinated, the sentence could read, "When the wound drained purulent material, the patient's temperature spiked to 103.2 degrees Fahrenheit."

Compound Sentences

A compound sentence has two or more independent clauses usually joined by "and," "but," "or," "nor," "for," "yet," or a semicolon. For example:

- The ICU nurse could not start an I.V., and a cutdown was necessary.
- The patient's pulse rate was fast, but it decreased 20 minutes after the patient took the medication.
- A care plan is essential; it guides consistent nursing care.

Use compound sentences when coordinate ideas are expressed in comparison, contrast, or balance: "The patient's pulse increased, but her blood pressure remained the same." Use a compound sentence when you want to give equal emphasis to two related ideas: "Costs must be cut; quality must be maintained."

Compound–Complex Sentences

A compound–complex sentence is created when a compound sentence contains dependent clauses, for example, "Based on the data from the needs assessment, a new course will be offered in budgeting for nurse managers, and the hemodynamic monitoring course will be offered on evening shift."

Compound–complex sentences tend to be longer than the other kinds of sentences. Use compound–complex sentences to show coordinate ideas, either or both of which are qualified.

Run-On Sentences

One additional problem about which editors commented was run-on sentences. Run-on sentences occur when two complete sentences are run together without any punctuation. A run-on sentence follows: "He experienced chest pain at the high altitude this alarmed the flight nurse." Correct the sentence by placing a period of semicolon after "altitude."

Check your manuscript to see if you have used variety in the types of sentences: simple, compound, complex, and compound–complex. Also check to see if any of the sentences are run-ons.

EMPHASIZING IDEAS

You will want to emphasize some ideas while you de-emphasize others. The following guidelines will help you to emphasize your ideas:

- *Put the idea in a simple sentence.* "She died."
- *Use active voice.* "Magnet hospitals are models of hospital nursing practice."
- *Place the idea at the beginning or end.* "An increase in the nurse-to-patient ratio was essential with the change in patient population on the unit."
- *Put the idea in a list.* "The job satisfaction survey showed nurses on the oncology unit 1) felt challenged; 2) appreciated positive feedback from patients; 3) did not want 10-hour shifts."
- *Use specific, concrete nouns to emphasize your idea.* "Nurses, physicians, a social worker, dietician, and physical therapist collaborated to plan the patient's discharge."
- *Use the idea as the subject of the sentence.* "Chemotherapeutic treatment for the patient's colon cancer was considered."
- *Use the command form.* "Examine the foot. Look at the x-rays."
- *Indicate that the idea is important.* "The most important facet of assessing

a snakebite victim is determining whether or not the reptile is poisonous"

- *Repeat the idea in different ways.* "An effective resume is one of your most valuable tools for professional advancement. Your resume helps you seize opportunities as they present themselves. Without an effective one, you may watch opportunities disappear" (Dowdney, 1984, p. 13).

VARIETY IN SENTENCES

To keep your writing interesting, use variety in beginning your sentences as well as in the kinds of sentences you write. The following are examples of different ways to begin sentences:

1. *Noun–verb:* "Consultation is a relatively new career opportunity for the registered nurse."
2. *Prepositional phrase:* "In the United States, tetanus most commonly results from puncture wounds of the extremities by nails or splinters contaminated with human or animal excreta."
3. *Adjective:* "Gigantic losses were anticipated."
4. *Adverb:* "Unfortunately, with a greater opportunity to play and compete, there is greater occurrence of sports-related injuries."
5. *Adverbial clause:* "When using shortened tracheostomy tubes, it is important to smooth the cut end of the tube and then to clean the tube before inserting it."
6. *Participial phrase:* "Introducing the suction catheter into the respiratory tract through the endotracheal tube bypasses the patient's normal upper airway defense mechanisms."
7. *Noun clause:* "That you can leave the clinic immediately after the acupuncture session is probable."
8. *Imperative:* "Read all the instructions about the procedure before you begin."
9. *Connective:* "However, many hospice programs fail to provide adequate training and support to volunteers."
10. *Transitional phrase:* "Furthermore, the situation needs to be viewed from another perspective."
11. *Question:* "Have you ever thought about circumcision? Why do we do it? Should we do it?"

Examine the beginnings of your sentences. When more than three consecutive sentences begin in the same way, change one of them to add variety to your writing. Then determine the sentence structures you typically use. Change some of the sentence structures to add variety to your writing.

SEXISM AND STEREOTYPES

Sexism and stereotypes in writing offend readers. Write about women and girls as having the same interests, abilities, and ambitions as men and boys. Florence Downs, Editor of *Nursing Research,* said:

> References to "man" in research articles appear with regularity. . . . Why this is so common has always been somewhat of a mystery to me, particularly in a profession that is predominantly female. One would think that this would be one of the last places this kind of sexist terminology cold be found. . . . From now on, let's write what we mean, human beings or an equivalent such as people. It is really not necessary to use the same term as that found in an original source, as long as the meaning remains unchanged. (1983, p. 195)

However, the problem is not always easily corrected. Edith Lewis (1976), in an editorial in *Nursing Outlook,* wrote, "It's a real editorial dilemma—one you can't win for losing. Use 'she' and you slight the men in the profession; use 'he' and you derogate the equality of women; use 'they' and individual nurses of both sexes are reduced to an amorphous blur; use 'he and/or she' and you are left with an awkward, graceless phrase" (p. 293).

Lewis concluded that the purpose of writing is to convey information in "as readable a fashion as possible," not to use language to fight the battle of the sexes. The writer's first obligation is to the reader, not to the writer "seeking, through artificial word usages, to rectify the social ills of the profession and the world" (Lewis, 1976, p. 293).

Although difficult to correct, stereotyped writing needs to be addressed because it exerts a powerful influence and limits the development of sex roles within a variety of occupations. You can avoid sexist writing by recasting passages in the plural and using "they," "them," and "their," or you can replace stereotypical terms by using nonsexist descriptions of occupations ("firefighter" for "fireman"). Be careful to use parallel terms. For example, instead of "man and wife," use "husband and wife."

The Handbook of Nonsexist Writing by Casey Miller and Kate Swift (1980) deals with this topic by presenting practical suggestions for those who are committed to equality as well as clarity in style. The authors use hundreds of examples that illustrate sexism in writing.

> Thoughtful efforts to avoid sexist phraseology through rewording rather than shortcuts such as s/he will probably yield some unexpected benefits. You are

likely to discover that the extra grooming will produce smoother sentence structure and a more accurate expression of the meaning you hope to convey, which, in the end, is what manuscript preparation is all about (Downs, 1983, p. 195).

Examine your manuscript for any sexist or stereotypical words or phrases.

DEHUMANIZING WORDS

Look for any examples of words or sentences that dehumanize people. Replace words that dehumanize people, such as "case" instead of "patient." Instead of saying "diabetics" or "schizophrenics," say "diabetic patient" or "a woman who is schizophrenic." Write "a man who is blind" rather than "blind man" or describe someone as comatose rather than as "a vegetable."

Put humanity into everything you write. Write about people. "Don't write about crop failures. Write about farmers in crisis. Don't write about romance. Write about people in love," said Gary Provost (1984b, p. 37).

Review your manuscript for dehumanizing terms and replace them.

VAGUE WORDS

Sometimes writers use vague rather than specific words, as in "We talked about a controversial issue." Who spoke:? What issue? "Roger and Barbara argued about collective bargaining for nurses," is more specific. It tells who was speaking, how they were speaking, and what issue was involved.

Vague words and phrases such as the following should be clarified: extremely, few, many, several, short, frequently, quite, vast, very, and some.

Replace every vague word or phrase in your manuscript with a specific, concrete one, if possible.

TRANSITIONS

Transitions lead readers from one section to another; they give manuscripts logic and cohesiveness. Transitions link sentences and paragraphs while providing a continuous thread of an idea through the manuscript. The reader's mind follows this thread, and you lose the reader if the thread is not continuous. Suzanne Hall Johnson (1993) also points out that "transition sentences also clarify a key point so that the reader can distinguish the main point from specific details in an article or book."

Some transitional phrases that may smooth out your manuscript are:
To indicate a summary statement: In summary, in brief, in short, in other words, in conclusion, or finally.

- *To indicate a result:* Hence, thus, therefore, accordingly, consequently, or as a result.
- *To indicate an additional thought:* Moreover, further, furthermore, also, too, in addition, first, second, third, etc.
- *To indicate a contrasting idea:* However, still, nevertheless, on the other hand, on the contrary, in contrast, or otherwise.
- *To indicate a comparison:* Similarly or likewise.
- *To illustrate:* For example, for instance, or to illustrate.
- *To show relationship to time:* At the same time, meanwhile, earlier, then, or next.

You can insert transitions to smooth your manuscript's flow. However, if you still do not achieve an even flow with transitions, you may be dealing with a different problem. Perhaps you need to eliminate an unrelated thought or reorder part of your manuscript. This requires a "cut and paste" approach—not stringing it together with transitions.

Be aware also of overuse of transitions. Edit out some if your manuscript reads "however . . . however . . . therefore . . . however."

Examine your manuscript to see if paragraphs are linked together so that one thought flows smoothly to the next. Insert transitions where they help to smooth the flow of thoughts.

HEADINGS

Headings can improve your reader's comprehension and interest because they summarize, emphasize, and outline ideas so that readers can follow your organization. They allow the reader to skim articles. To use headings appropriately, consult the publication's writer's guidelines or analyze current article issues to see how the publication uses headings.

Look at the Sun Diagram you prepared before you wrote your manuscript. See if the individual rays are actually headings for the manuscript.

PARALLEL STRUCTURE

Parallel structure pulls related ideas together through repeating similar grammatical patterns. For example, "The ways to grow professionally include (1) reading professional publications; (2) discussing current topics with colleagues; and (3) attending professional seminars, workshops, and conferences."

The first word following a number in the above list is in parallel grammatical structure. Thus, parallel grammatical structure requires ideas that are similar in content, function, and importance to be expressed in similar form. The key in using parallelism correctly is being consistent in verb tense, person, voice, and grammatical structure.

Rewrite sentences that are without parallel grammatical structure. For instance, examine the following unparallel sentence: "Nurses play multiple roles as teachers, taking care of patients, and they do management." You can rewrite this sentence in parallel form in several ways: "Nurses play multiple roles: they are teachers, clinicians, and managers." Or: "Nurses play multiple roles—teaching students, caring for patients, and managing other nurses." Or: "Nurses function in educational, clinical, and management roles." Or: "Nurses are educators, clinicians, and managers." These examples offer a wide range of approaches to conveying equivalent ideas in parallel form.

If you listed items in your manuscript, check the list to ensure that the first word in each listing is in the same parallel grammatical structure.

JARGON AND CLICHES

Jargon consists of a group of words used primarily by members of a particular professional, social, or other group. Jargon may "sacrifice efficiency and precision for a long-winded, flabby vagueness" (Sears, 1979, p. 25).

Examples of words that could be considered jargon include: Conceptual model, crisis intervention, behavioral objective, paradigm, frame-of-reference, ombudsman, logistics, cost-containment, ping-ponging, overview, quantify, private sector, public sector, etc.

Although using jargon may be an easy way out of a difficult writing situation, Ellen Goldensohn said:

> Don't resort to jargon just because you're a bit too tired to find the word that's just right. . . . If you feel an irresistible craving to use jargon, implement the appropriate prophylactic interventions to optimize and enhance your verbalization utilization skill. Don't give in. Remember, better red than erythematous (Goldensohn, 1982, p. 541).

In *The Book of Jargon* (Miller, 1981), a collection of jargon from diverse groups, the author wrote that the language of the medical profession is almost a foreign language: "Medicalese characteristically describes patients in terms of their disorders and their (diseased) organs and parts. . . . The language reflects the profession's tendency to regard the magnificent and complex human being as a machine. . . . This depersonalized professionalism is established and sustained effectively through the use of medical terminology and jargon" (pp. 3–4). The nursing profession shares some of this problem.

Cliches are also to be avoided in writing. Write them during your free flow writing to hold the idea. Then search for a more specific way to replace them during your editing. Gary Provost wrote,

> I've just finished a book called *One Hundred Ways to Improve Your Writing*. Way #75 was "Avoid Cliches." I wrote: Cliches are a dime a dozen. If you've seen one you've seen them all. They've been used once too often. They've outlived their usefulness. Their familiarity breeds contempt. They make the writer look dumb as a doornail, and they cause the reader to sleep like a log. So be sly as a fox. Avoid cliches like the plague. If you start to use one, drop it like a hot potato. Instead, be as smart as a whip. Write something that is fresh as a daisy, cute as a button and sharp as a tack. Better safe than sorry. (Provost, 1984, p. 36)

Examine your manuscript for jargon and cliches, and replace them with more effective and appropriate words.

PUNCTUATION

Although the purpose of most punctuation is the same—to group some words and to separate others—the various marks differ in degree. Commas show some separation, semicolons more, and periods the most. Dashes reflect more of a separation than commas but less than parentheses. Dashes and parentheses interrupt. Colons show connection and anticipation. Semicolons mark a break or contrast.

If punctuation is a problem in your writing, consult *The Chicago Manual of Style* published by the University of Chicago Press (1993), *The Publication Manual of the American Psychological Association* (1994) or Scientific Style and Format (Council of Biology Editors, 1994).

READABILITY

Readability formulas indicate the difficulty of written material according to the skill or school grade level needed to understand it. Several formulas have been developed that help writers use the most appropriate reading level for a particular audience. Many computer software programs will generate readability reports.

IMPROVING YOUR WRITING

Consider the following principles for improving your writing:

1. Be concise. Omit all unnecessary words, phrases, and ideas.
2. Be specific. Avoid generalizations.
3. Use the active voice whenever possible.
4. Use strong verbs rather than smothered verbs.
5. Use the simple, familiar word rather than the long or obscure word.
6. Organize the manuscript logically.
7. Use headings to guide your reader.
8. Use parallel structure in lists and sentences.
9. State your purpose clearly.

Table 9.2. Checklist for Revision (© 1995, Dowdney & Sheridan)

❐ Headings consistent in placement and grammatical form
❐ Transitions between paragraphs clearly linking one idea to the next
❐ Variety in sentence beginnings
❐ Variety in sentence types
❐ Variety in sentence length
❐ No sexist, stereotypical or dehumanizing terms
❐ No unnecessary words and phrases
❐ No over-reliance on passive voice
❐ Concrete words
❐ Clear pronoun reference
❐ No jargon
❐ Abbreviating or acronyms explained
❐ Correct spelling
❐ No confusing or awkward sentences
❐ Numbers and facts accurate
❐ Consistent capitalization and punctuation
❐ Sentences understandable
❐ Interesting information
❐ Significant information
❐ Believable information
❐ Clear connection between beginning and ending
❐ Correct and complete references

Careful editing of your manuscript allows you to write freely, knowing that you will clean it up later. Each time you edit your manuscripts you will become more aware of your specific rewriting needs.

As you use the Checklist for Revision (Table 9.2) to edit your manuscript, you may find it useful to use proofreader's marks. Many dictionaries include proofreader's marks along with a sample marked copy. You will need to understand these symbols when edited copy is returned from your editor.

Your edited copy is ready for review from your colleagues, final preparation, and presentation to the editor. Chapter Ten addresses these final steps.

EXERCISE

Review your manuscript once more by using the Checklist for Revision.

REFERENCES

American Psychological Association. (1994). *Publication manual of the American Psychological Association* (4th ed.). Washington, DC: Author.

Castledine, G. (1982, June). A poor record in writing. *Nursing Mirror, 154*(6), 31.

Council of Biology Editors. (1994). *Scientific style and format.* New York: Cambridge University Press.

Curtin, L. (1981). The jawbone of an ass. *Supervisor Nurse, 12*(7), 7.

Dowdney, D. (1984). For professional advancement: Your resume. *Nursing Management, 15*(8), 13–14.

Dowdney, D. L., & Sheridan, D. R. (1984). Survey of nursing and health care journal editors. (Unpublished work).

Downs, F. (1983). S/He. *Nursing Research, 32*(4), 195.

Goldensohn, E. (1982, November–December). Acute fulminating jargonitis. *Nursing Outlook, 9,* 541.

Johnson, S. H. (1993). *Nurse author.* Writing transition sentences. 3(4), 8–9.

Lewis, E. (1974). Pretentious prose. *Nursing Outlook, 22*(7), 431.

Lewis, E. (1976). Whither he and/or she going? *Nursing Outlook, 24*(5), 293.

Miller, C., & Swift, K. (1980). *The handbook of nonsexist writing.* New York: Lippincott & Crowell.

Miller, D. E. (1981). *The book of jargon.* New York: Macmillan.

Provost, G. (1984a, May). Ain't you a little too concerned about perfect English? *Writer's Digest,* p. 20.

Provost, G. (1984b, March). Beacons of excellent writing. *Writer's Digest,* p. 37.

Provost, G. (1984c, October). The perfect match. *Writer's Digest,* p. 36.

Schwager, E. (1991). *Medical English usage and abusage* (pp. 41–42). Phoenix: Oryx.

Sears, J. (1979, September). Jargon and gobbledygook. A checklist of symptoms. *The American Business Communication Association Bulletin, 42*(3), 25–27.

Strunk, W., & White, E. B. (1979). *The elements of style.* New York: Macmillan.

University of Chicago Press. (1993). *The Chicago manual of style* (13th ed.). Chicago: Author.

Zinsser, W. (1980). *On writing well.* New York: Harper & Row.

10

Prepare and Send the Manuscript

Sit down, relax, and carefully read through the revised draft of your manuscript once again. Evaluate it for overall format and content. Then test it on your colleagues.

FORMAT

Format is a manuscript's physical arrangement and general appearance. Good formats help readers understand your ideas. Check the journal's format requirements to ensure that your manuscript complies with its guidelines. Did you write a manuscript that is congruent with the analysis you prepared of your target journal?

Manuscript styles vary considerably in specifications for headings, titles, figures, tables, lists of references, and other manuscript features. Editorial styles have been established by many professional organizations such as the American Chemical Society, American Medical Association, American Psychological Association (APA), American Sociological Association, Council of Biology Editors, Modern Language Association, University of Chicago, and the U.S. Government Printing Office. In nursing the APA style is frequently used.

Some formats require inclusion of the following: abstract; title page; headings; references; and illustrative materials. The following pages describe these format elements.

Abstract

Abstracts condense large pieces of writing into 100 to 300 words. Abstracts highlight and summarize the manuscript's major points and state the facts on which conclusions are based.

> Because the Abstract precedes the paper itself, and because the editors and reviewers like a bit of orientation, the Abstract is almost universally the first part of the manuscript read during the review process. Therefore, it is of fundamental importance that the Abstract be written clearly and simply. If you cannot attract the interest of the reviewer in your Abstract, your cause may be lost. Very often, the reviewer may be perilously close to a final judgment of your manuscript after reading the Abstract alone. (Day, 1994, p. 31)

Three of the most common types of abstracts are the annotative abstract—an explanatory note indicating the major purpose or theme of the article; the indicative abstract, which provides general information amplifying the title; and the informative abstract, which gives the readers as complete a summary as possible (Robinson & Notter, 1982).

> An abstract is a brief, comprehensive summary of the contents of the article; it allows readers to survey the contents of an article quickly and, like a title, is used by abstracting and information services to index and retrieve articles. . . . A well-prepared abstract can be the most important paragraph in your article. . . . Most people will have their first contact with an article by seeing just the abstract, usually on a computer screen with several other abstracts, as they are doing a literature search through an electronic abstract-retrieval system. Readers frequently decide on the basis of the abstract whether to read the entire article; this is true whether the reader is at a computer or is thumbing through a journal. The abstract needs to be dense with information but also readable, well organized, brief, and self-contained. Also, embedding many key words in your abstract will enhance the user's ability to find it. A good abstract is accurate . . . self-contained . . . concise and specific . . . nonevaluative . . . coherent and readable. (American Psychological Association, 1994, pp. 8–9)

Some nursing publications request authors to follow the American Medical Association (AMA) *Manual of Style*. For example, the *Journal of Nursing Administration's* writer's guidelines state, "Unless otherwise stated here, prepare manuscripts according to the American Medical Association (AMA) Manual of Style. (8th edition)" (Information for authors, 1993, p. 70).

If you are writing an abstract of a research paper, include "statements of the problem, method, results, and conclusions. An abstract of a review or theoretical article should state the topics covered, the organizing idea, the sources used (e.g., personal observation, published literature, or previous research bearing on the topic), and the conclusions drawn" (Gelderman, 1984, p. 45).

Do not write an abstract until after you have completed your manuscript. Then begin with the manuscript's topic sentence and summarize the most important topics through reviewing any headings. As you do this, eliminate all unnecessary details.

When you write an abstract, use the following guidelines:

- Summarize the contents of articles.
- Do not include anything that is not in the article.
- Define all key abbreviations and acronyms.
- Paraphrase rather than quote information.
- Do not include references or illustrations.
- Reflect the article correctly (do not add your opinions or evaluations).
- Present information concisely and coherently.
- Indicate the problem or question investigated.
- State the method used.
- Give the results, conclusions, or implications.

Abstracts can help indexers in preparing indexes for articles and can help reference librarians in retrieving relevant articles. They assist translators in preparing information for foreign readers. Abstracts helps readers judge the value of articles. They also facilitate electronic searches of databases.

Title Page

Because each journal uses a preferred style for article title pages, consult the journal's guidelines. Most journals require the names and degrees of all authors; other styles omit all job titles.

If the research for your manuscript received funding from a supporting agency, foundation, fellowship, scholarship, or internship, some publications require that you present this information in a specified manner. Check with the source of your grant for attribution requirements, and review the grant recognition format the journal specifies.

Headings

Headings guide readers through manuscripts by dividing information into manageable segments, signaling topic changes, indicating the manuscript's organization, and establishing each topic's importance. Every topic of equal importance must have the same level of heading through-out the manuscript. Because headings also indicate a shift to a new topic or subtopic, prepare all headings with the same parallel grammatical structure so that all sentence elements that are alike in function are also alike in construction.

In long, complex manuscripts, you may need several levels of headings to indicate divisions, subdivisions, and other units. Consult the journal's writer's guidelines to determine appropriate heading choices.

References

Reference citations document the statements in the text. All citations in the manuscript must appear in the reference list; all references must be cited in text. Place the reference list at the end of your manuscript unless the journal's writer's guidelines specify otherwise.

Be sure that you look at your target journal and that you copy the reference style exactly as you prepare your manuscript. Although not reason by itself for rejection, editors find incomplete reference citations and citations not in the journal's format annoying.

Illustrative Materials

Illustrative materials such as tables, graphs, and photographs aid readers in absorbing a manuscript's ideas.

> Each table should be self-explanatory, present one point leading to a single conclusion, be accurate, and contain only data relevant to the purpose of the table. In general, a description of what the table offers comes from reading the table's title, column heads and subs, and footnotes. (Lister, 1981, p. 1803)

Good illustrations convey ideas that words alone cannot make clear; they can enrich your manuscript.

> Decide whether illustrations are necessary to complete the written word and which ideas need pictorial assistance. If a written description is liable to leave readers confused or a picture can save lengthy explanation, illustrate the technique, position, equipment, or anatomical structure. Generally, convey one thought for one illustration. But be economical, too. Many authors are able to refer to the same figure several times throughout an article. . . . Illustrate only what needs depiction; delete unnecessary details that could confuse or mislead readers. (George, 1981, p. 1489)

Do not use illustrations as decorations; they must supplement your article's information. Do not use so many illustrations that you distract readers from the article's content.

When illustrations are presented with clarity and consistency, they help readers focus on key portions of manuscripts. Use the following guidelines adapted from *Handbook of Technical Writing* (Brusaw, 1993) to plan your manuscript's illustrations:

- Keep illustrations brief and simple.
- Present only one type of information in each illustration.
- Label or write a caption for each illustration.
- Include an identification key for all symbols.
- Specify the proportions you used.
- Use horizontal lettering.
- Use consistent terminology in the text and illustrations.
- Leave white space around and within the illustration.
- Place the illustration close to the text to which it refers; illustrations usually do not appear ahead of the first text reference to them.
- Make the significance of each illustration clear.
- Make figure or table numbers consecutive.

If you have access to a computer and a good software graphics program, try creating graphics on the computer. The results are astounding as numerical data print as pie, bar, line, or area graphs. Some computer programs prepare even more elaborate graphic presentations of data. Computer graphics are especially useful if you are writing for journals with administrative, economic, financial, or research themes.

PREPARING THE FINAL DRAFT

Type the manuscript on one side of plain, 20-pound bond white paper. Avoid using the erasable or onionskin paper because type on these kinds of paper smears onto the reader's fingers and off the paper. Use plain white paper rather than colored paper or paper with a border.

Editors need room in the margins for their comments. Use the margins that the writer's guidelines specify. If no guidelines are given, leave at least 1½" on all sides. If you have a word processor that is capable of justifying the margins (spacing the words so that the lines end as evenly on the right side of the paper as on the left), do not use this feature. Editors need to estimate words in various sections of the manuscript, and justified margins hinder the word counting process.

Use pica (10-pitch) type if possible; elite (12-pitch) is also acceptable, but avoid exotic or script typestyles or typestyles that capitalize all letters. These are difficult to read and look "cute" rather than professional. Place your title and page number at the top corners of each page so that if the pages become separated, the editor can reassemble the manuscript easily.

Use a paper clip on the upper left corner of the manuscript rather than stapling it together or binding it in a cover. A fancy cover or leather binding containing a manuscript shows the editor that an amateur writer has sent the manuscript.

If you need to make any last-minute changes, you are fortunate if the manuscript is in a word processor's memory because the pages can be retyped quickly. Using a regular typewriter, you may be able to retype parts of the pages with changes, using white-out, cut-and-paste, or photocopy, but be sure to send a clean copy. Retype any page entirely, if necessary, for good quality.

COPYRIGHT AND PERMISSIONS

Copyright

Copyright is a statutory grant to a copyright owner giving exclusive rights over the use of the material. The 1976 Omnibus Copyright Revision Act provides protection for works created after January 1, 1978 for a term lasting the author's lifetime, plus an additional 50 years after the author's death. Works already protected under the old law will now be covered for a maximum of 75 years (this consists of a 28-year period, plus a renewal). These rights are transferred to the journal when you sign their contract.

Review recent journal issues to determine the journal's copyright policy. Most nurses assign full rights to the publishing company, and the contract the company sends you for your signature is a standard practice. You can try to negotiate to give "first rights" only, but since all editors want new material, your chances of using it again in a health care journal are almost nonexistent. It may also cause the editor to wonder whether your currently submitted manuscript has been previously published. If you want to write on this topic again, you would need to write a new article for the target journal.

The only restriction on the monopoly given to the copyright holder is the recognition that the public at large is entitled to make "fair use" of a copyrighted work for certain purposes and within reasonable limits, provided due credit is given. There is no hard line between fair and unfair use. In practice, the borrower must decide in which category his or her particular intended use falls. The *Chicago Manual of Style* (1993) suggests considering the following factors in determining fair use:

1. The purpose and character of the use, including whether such use is of a commercial nature or is for nonprofit educational purposes.
2. The nature of the copyrighted work.
3. The amount and substantiality of the portion used in relation to the copyrighted work as a whole.
4. The effect of the use upon the potential market for, or value of, the copyrighted work (p. 146).

The following questions may help you to assess fair use:

1. *What is the length of the extract relative to the length of the work?* A quotation of 200 words from a 2,000-word article would not be fair use, whereas 500 words from a 500-page book would probably be fair. One should also note the combined length of several short extracts from the same source. If the combined length would not comprise fair use in a connected quote of the same length, permission should be sought.

2. *What is the importance of the extract relative to the entire work?* It is not length alone that is critical, but also the significance of the part to the whole. Generally, anything used in its entirety (such as an article, chapter, table, or figure) would not be considered fair use.

3. *Can the extract serve as a substitute for the original?* Would reprinting it affect the sales or profitability of the original?

There are some instances in which determining fair use is more straightforward. Unpublished writings are not in the public domain; there is no provision for fair use, and permission should always be obtained from the author. On the other hand, publications of the U.S. government are not copyrighted and may be used freely. Note however, that material previously copyrighted does not lose its copyright by being included in a government publication.

Permissions

Permissions involve granting either an author or a publisher the right to excerpt copyrighted material for use within another work. Authors are responsible for obtaining permission to quote or copy material. As early as possible in the manuscript preparation stage, design a form similar to Figure 10.1 for obtaining permissions from copyright holders. Give exact identification of what and how much material you will be using. Specify pages,

Date:
To: (Full name and address of publisher)
From: (Your name and address)
Re: Request for Permission to Publish

I would like to reprint the following material from your publication (State the exact information to identify the material.)

Description: _____

Author: _____

Title: _____

Edition: _____

City: _____

Publisher: _____

Publication date: _____

In considering this request, please note that I intend to use this material in (name of your new publication). Please sign and return one copy of this letter and retain one for your files. I am enclosing a stamped, addressed envelope. I appreciate your consideration of this request.

Sincerely,

(Your signature)

We grant permission for publication as stated above. Credit will be given as follows unless you specify otherwise:

Signature: _____

Name (printed):   _____

Date: _____

Figure 10.1. Request for Permission Form (© 1995, Dowdney & Sheridan).

number of paragraphs, number of words, and whether you plan to include illustrations. Make a photocopy of the material you want to use and highlight the specifics for clarity. Attach the photocopy to your form and refer to it on the Permissions Form. Include whatever is relevant and whatever might serve to forestall a request from the copyright holder for more precise information. This will save you unnecessary correspondence. Describe your intended use as clearly as possible. Sometimes copyright holders will lower or waive a fee if they understand that the material is to be used in a scholarly journal rather than in one for a general audience. If you are requesting permission to reprint from a journal, check a recent issue to find out what the permission policy is. This too can save extra correspondence.

The Literary Market Place, a paperbound work published yearly, contains publishers' addresses and, in many cases, the name of the person in charge of granting permissions. Be sure to send each copyright holder two copies of your letter, one for the holder's files and one to sign and return to you.

It is crucial that *all* stipulations of the copyright holder be met. Thus, if a publisher requires that you obtain permission from the author, do not neglect to do so. If a form is to be filled in and returned, do so promptly.

Some users are inclined to write for permission from the author and the publisher simultaneously. This is not advisable because it doubles correspondence and causes delays. Authors are harder to locate than publishers. If the publisher requires that the author's permission be obtained, you may ask the publisher for the author's most recent address.

Occasionally you may have difficulty in determining who (if anyone) holds copyright on a work. It is never safe to assume that a book is in the public domain because it is out of print, no one answers your letter requesting permission to reprint, the author is dead, the publisher is no longer in business, or no descendants or heirs of the author can be located.

If you are unclear about the copyright status of a work, write to the Register of Copyrights, Washington, D.C. 20025, for a search of the records. A fee is charged for this service. Although the Register's failure to turn up a copyright record is not conclusive evidence that none exists, an official reply is a token of your good faith in attempting to establish copyright status.

Keep track of the permissions you request. Be sure that all stipulations have been or will be met prior to publication. Keep copies of your permission request forms. Send completed forms to your editor.

Credit lines as printed in a publication represent the copyright holder's protection against infringement of his or her rights as owner. It is crucial that a requested credit line be followed word for word and symbol for symbol. If the publisher's permission does not specify a particular wording, the credit line should be in the form of the following example:

- *Book:* Donna Richards Sheridan; Jean Eppinger Bronstein; and Duane D. Walker. *The New Nurse Manager: A Guide to Management Development.* Copyright © 1984 by Aspen Systems Corporation, Gaithersburg, MD. Reprinted by permission of the publisher.
- *Journal:* Donna Lee Dowdney: "For Professional Advancement: Your Resume." Copyright © 1984 by *Nursing Management.* Reprinted by permission of the publisher.

Fill in the credit line on the Permissions Form prior to sending it (See Figure 10.1). The publisher can change it if desired.

It is important to remember that requesting permission unnecessarily is not advisable; you may become involved in extensive, tedious correspondence that could delay your manuscript's production. This does not mean, of course, that the source of short quotes should not be clearly credited in footnotes or the bibliography. If you are preparing a manuscript that makes extensive use of copyrighted material, you can find useful, detailed information on permissions in *A Manual of Style* (University of Chicago Press, 1993).

Fees

The author is responsible for paying fees for obtaining permissions. If a grantor insists on a very high fee for material that you need to use, discuss the problem with your editor *before* signing any agreement to pay, or reconsider how important that information is to your article.

GLOSSARY

A glossary is a list of terms that you select, define, and explain. It usually appears at a manuscript's conclusion or as a sidebar. If you write materials for people who are unfamiliar with specialized terms in your manuscript, then consider preparing a glossary.

One way to decide which words to incorporate in a glossary is to have someone who is unfamiliar with your specialized area read your manuscript and underline all unfamiliar terms. Then place each term on an index card and define it. Next, alphabetize the terms and add them to the manuscript's glossary. It is not necessary to define technical or scientific terms for a technical or scientific journal designed for specialists. However, a glossary is always useful if nonspecialists will refer to your manuscript.

CONTENT

After being intensely involved in writing an article, you may find it difficult to review it objectively. However, you might try the following: As you read your manuscript once more, imagine that you have never previously seen it. Pretend that you are on a break at work and that you begin skimming a journal on the lounge table. As you look at the title you selected, do you know the manuscript's content immediately?

As you turn to the page on which you imagine your article appearing, is it visually appealing because it is divided into enough paragraphs and headings to present content in a visually appealing manner? Long, uninterrupted text is unappealing to readers. Read the first line or two. Does it have a hook? Does it draw you into the article?

If you wrote an abstract, read it again to see if it represents the content accurately and is interesting. Could the abstract stand alone on a library search or computer printout as an accurate representation of your article?

Now read the article in the way you read most journal articles. If you typically read slowly and thoughtfully, read it this way. If you are a quick reader and skim articles, do that now. Watch for any points that cause you to "wade" through the material or places that tempt your mind to wander. These points may need clarification, or perhaps you need to tighten up the text with some brutal editing. Are there places where the article seems to superficially skim the content?

Watch for "bumps." If you are reading along and something bothers you, check for changes in tense or needed transitions. Look for value statements and consider possible implications of what you have said. Decide if you enjoy the article and whether your colleagues would enjoy it. Would you find this information useful? What would make this article more enjoyable or interesting?

REACTIONS FROM YOUR COLLEAGUES

After you write several drafts, ask your colleagues to read your manuscript. Do not skip this vital step, even if you are tempted to hurry through the Writing Process. You do not want your manuscript to create controversy because of incorrect or unclear data—especially if negative clinical consequences are possible. For instance, check drug dosages carefully. Other errors that surface to haunt you could include inaccurate quotations, incorrectly spelled words, or improper use of a theory or framework.

Verify all facts in your manuscript. In the event that you miss something, ask respected colleagues in your field to provide the careful second look that your manuscript may need. Feedback from your colleagues serves as a barometer to help you determine if others understand your manuscript. Through their feedback you will obtain a better sense of the manuscript's appropriateness and effectiveness. Feedback helps you identify unclear words or incomplete thoughts.

Your colleagues may not feel comfortable giving you anything but positive feedback. This is because sometimes, in asking for feedback, authors give a strong secondary message such as "I hope you like this," or "I've really worked hard on this." What these authors are seeking is encouragement. While everyone needs encouragement in learning new skills, that message does not result in useful recommendations. Instead, it keeps your colleagues from giving you anything but positive feedback.

Nurses have asked us what to do when they are asked to review manuscripts that are poorly organized. The type of input you need from a colleague addresses timeliness, content (for example, clinical correctness), format, and appropriate reference citations. Although it is difficult to give negative feedback, your colleague needs and is seeking this input. Be sure to include a positive feedback. Criticism, or negative feedback, should be given as suggestions.

We designed the Manuscript Critique Form (Figure 10.2) so that you may copy it and give it to your colleagues when you ask them to review your manuscripts. The form gives a clear message about what you want and that you value honest criticism. It also arranges comments in a format that is easy to use.

Select three people to give you feedback: a nurse in your field, a nurse not in your field, and a non-nurse. If this third person is a writing expert, it would be especially helpful because that person approaches the manuscript with writing expertise and without any bias or prejudice about the topic, or knowledge of specialized jargon. This person may review the manuscript with more objectivity than your colleagues could give it. You can hire an editor to review your manuscript and use the feedback to learn more about your writing strengths and weaknesses. This, however, does not replace the input you need from other nurses.

Consider each suggestion seriously. Try to understand what is behind the feedback. Do not be so wedded to your work that you cannot change words, phrases, thoughts, and sequences for improved clarity. Nevertheless, you have the final decision about what you will write and how you will write it.

You also might want to initiate a manuscript critique group. Rather than being a mutual admiration society that praises each other's manuscripts, you would meet to encourage and assist each other in preparing good manuscripts. A few guidelines for a manuscript critique group include the following:

Dear Colleague,

I am asking you to review the attached manuscript because of your expertise. As you read, please note in the manuscript's margins any points that are unclear or incorrect as well as any grammatical or spelling errors. When you have finished, please complete the questions below. Thank you.

Manuscript title _____

Date needed _____

Targeted journal(s)

_____

_____

1. Do you consider the manuscript
☐ timely
☐ interesting
☐ organized
☐ readable
☐ important

2. Did anything in the manuscript "talk down," "talk over your head" or offend you? If yes, please explain._____

_____

_____

3. What did you like best about the manuscript?

_____

_____

_____

4. What is the weakest point? How can I improve the manuscript?_____

_____

_____

5. Please add additional suggestions and comments:

_____

_____

Figure 10.2. Manuscript Critique Form (© 1995, Dowdney & Sheridan).

- Set time limits for each writer's manuscript to be read. This is essential in preventing one individual from dominating the session. (Or schedule one manuscript per session.)
- Allow each writer to read a manuscript without interruption, questions, or lengthy explanations. (Or provide the manuscript to participants before the session so they can read it in advance.)
- Offer constructive comments for improving the manuscript and on selecting additional target markets.
- Evaluate the manuscript for clarity, style, structure, content, grammatical accuracy, and contribution to the nursing profession.

REFEREED PUBLICATIONS AND EDITORIAL REVIEW

Referees are "anonymous experts who are called upon to advise editors on the suitability of papers for publication" (Bishop, 1984, p. 45). The topic of writing for refereed or nonrefereed publications is a controversial one in nursing. Consider the significance of publishing in "refereed" journals and the importance of the refereed journal to the professsion's development, as you decide whether or not to publish in refereed journals.

> The attitude that refereed journals are better than non-refereed journals limits research dissemination. . . . Circulation statistics show that most nurses depend on one of three journals (*RN, American Journal of Nursing,* and *Nursing*) for their continuing education. Nurse researchers and nurse educators who wish to bring new knowledge to clinicians must therefore publish in these journals. That is unlikely to happen, however, until the academic rewards for promotion and tenure change. Nursing has been, in our opinion, overly quick to accept the distinction between refereed journals and non-refereed journals.

The authors went on to say:

> We contend that the nursing research community should stop valuing publication in refereed journals to the exclusion of others. Instead of judging research by the journal in which it is reported, we believe it is far better to judge research by its quality and significance. It *is* necessary to publish for and be evaluated by one's peers, but it is also necessary to publish so the practicing nurse can understand and have easy access to nursing research. (McCloskey & Buckwalter, 1982, pp. 255–256).

Donna Sheridan, who has served on several nursing editorial boards and reviewed many manuscripts, has found some manuscripts needed peer review or extensive editorial rework. This is especially true in attempts at humor that are actually put-downs, which are especially problematic in a profession that is addressing image issues. On the other hand, as a writer, Sheridan had one editor write to her about her own manuscript saying that although peer input suggested the article was too critical of nursing, "However, I've decided to publish it as is." There is much subjectivity even in those journals pursuing the referee process.

In addition, the referee process differs from journal to journal, adding to the controversy. If refereeing, each journal must decide how many, who should review, what should be reviewed, and how much impact the review should have.

Nursing Administration Quarterly uses editorial board review to determine the scholarly merit of articles.

All manuscripts are reviewed by at least two members of the editorial board. Members of the board evaluate manuscripts based on the following criteria:

- Concise, logical ordering of ideas
- Sound argument and defense of original ideas
- Accuracy of content
- Adequacy of documentation
- Use of sound methods of research or other forms of scholarly investigation
- Consistency with the purpose of the journal (*Nursing Administration Quarterly*, 1985)

These functions may also be performed by editors (often nurses) of nonrefereed journals.

Dimensions of Critical Care Nursing (DCCN) is a refereed journal; every article submitted is scrutinized by at least three expert reviewers. Michael Boyette, developmental editor of *DCCN*, described the review process:

When the editor receives your manuscript, she will first select three reviewers for your article. These reviewers, chosen from among the *DCCN* Editorial Board members and editorial consultants, are matched when possible to the subject matter of the article. For example, an article on a respiratory technique would be sent to a respiratory clinical nurse specialist; one on continuing education would be sent to an experienced critical care inservice educator; while an administrative article would be sent to a critical care nursing administrator. (Boyette, 1982, p. 375)

Boyette then indicated that the publication sends reviewers copies of articles with the names of authors removed to ensure objectivity. *DCCN* also does not reveal the names of reviewers to authors. Although criteria vary from journal to journal, the overall criteria sought by nurse editors is similar.

RETURN TO THE REVISION CHAPTER

After you receive peer or editor revision suggestions, if you see that you need to make a major revision, return to the previous chapter. If the manuscript's organization is the problem, return to your Sun Diagram and revise it, or construct several more diagrams until your material is well organized. Work back through the process. If the content is superficial, return to the library; then show the revised manuscript to your colleagues once again. You may need to return once more to the Sun Diagram to reorganize it. You may even need to return to the Writing Plan and rework it. If so, do not consider your first efforts in vain—writing is a process. Although we have helped make the process more linear to facilitate your writing, in actuality the process is cyclic as represented by feedback loops on the Model. Each time through any part of the cycle will clarify your thoughts and improve your manuscript.

SENDING YOUR MANUSCRIPT

Send a transmittal letter with your manuscript stating that you are enclosing the manuscript that the editor is expecting. Be sure to save a copy of your manuscript in the event it goes astray in the mail.

Place the manuscript and transmittal letter in a file folder to protect the manuscript. Address a 9 x 12 inch envelope to yourself and place adequate postage on it for first class delivery, for the manuscript's return. Then address a 10 x 13 inch envelope to the appropriate editor and mark the envelope first class, or send it through a delivery service such as Federal Express if you are enclosing timely materials. Next, enter the date sent in the comments column of the Manuscript Tracking Form.

Nursing 95 provided the following guidelines for sending manuscripts on paper as well as on disk.

> If possible, please send us your article on computer disk (in WordPerfect or an ASCII file), along with three printouts. If this isn't possible, submit your manuscript typed and double-spaced on standard-size typewriter paper, leaving generous margins so editors can make notes.
>
> Start with a cover page including your name, address, and home and work phone numbers. Be sure each page of your manuscript is numbered and

includes the title of your article. Don't put your name on each page, as we'd have to delete it before sending your article for a blind peer review. If there are multiple authors, please designate one to handle all contact with us. On separate pages, please include a single copy of each of the following:

- A list of references you used in preparing the article (none more than 5 years old, please).
- A brief description of your professional education and your present employer and position.
- A signed statement that no other publisher is considering your article and that you won't send it to another publisher until you hear from *Nursing*.

Include charts, illustrations, and photographs, if appropriate. Label and caption them clearly, and note the source if it's not your original creation. We will have illustrations redrawn by professional artists, but you may want to submit rough drawings that you feel would be helpful. We require signed releases from all persons photographed (we can supply forms if needed).

EXERCISES

1. Ask three peers to critique your manuscript, using the Manuscript Critique Form, and revise accordingly.
2. Prepare and send your manuscript.

REFERENCES

American Psychological Association. (1994). *Publication manual of the American Psychological Association* (4th ed.). Washington, DC: Author.

Bishop, C. (1984). *How to edit a scientific journal*. Philadelphia: ISI Press.

Boyette, M. (1982). The *DCCN* review process. *Dimensions of Critical Care Nursing, 1*(6), 375–378.

Brusaw, C. T., Alred, G. J., & Oliu, W. E. (1993). *Handbook of technical writing* (pp. 310–313). New York: St. Martin's Press.

Day, R. A. (1994). *How to write and publish a scientific paper*. Phoenix, AZ: Oryx.

Gelderman, C. (1984). *Better writing for professionals*. Glenview, IL: Scott Foresman.

George, S. (1981). Talking pictures. *Physical Therapy, 61*(10), 1489.

Information for authors. (1993). *Journal of Nursing Administration, 23*(9), 70.

Lister, M. (1981). Tables and figures. *Physical Therapy, 61*(12), 1803.

Literary Market Place. (Annual). New York: Bowker.

McCloskey, J. C., & Buckwalter, K. C. (1982). Publishing in non-refereed journals is not only O.K.—It's necessary. *Western Journal of Nursing Research, 4*(3), 255–256.

Nursing 95. (1995). Writer's guidelines for *Nursing 95.* [On-line]. Available: Guidelines, 73751, 42.

Nursing Administration Quarterly. (1985). *Author guide.* Rockville, MD: Aspen Systems Corp.

Robinson, A. M., & Notter, L. E. (1982). *Clinical writing for health professionals.* Bowie, MD: Robert J. Brady Co.

University of Chicago Press. (1995). *The Chicago manual of style* (14th ed.). Chicago, IL: Author.

Epilogue

Now that you have learned to use The Writing Process, you will never need to face a blank sheet of paper with dread. Instead you can be confident as you use The Writing Process to move forward from your initial idea to a published manuscript.

You have learned how to generate ideas for articles, overcome writer's block and use free-flow writing to write fast. You have also learned to identify your desired readers, along with their setting and specialty. You have discovered topics on which nursing journal editors would like to see articles. You have learned traditional ways to gather information as well as ways to use the new computerized information retrieval and transmission techniques. You have learned how to initiate communication with editors, and how to be your own editor so that you can revise your own manuscripts. You have gleaned insights from successful nurse authors about their writing experiences that may be helpful to you. You have learned to use a Plan and a Process to manage your writing tasks. You have seen examples of various writing frameworks and learned about organization.

Always recognize the importance of developing an article for a specific market by communicating effectively with journal editors. Use the skills you have learned to write fast, edit well, and prepare a quality manuscript—the kind of manuscript an editor enjoys receiving.

Rejection of your manuscript is unlikely at this stage if you have received a positive response to your query and sent a quality manuscript in a reasonable amount of time. However, if your manuscript is rejected you will probably receive information from the editor as to why. If not, ask. Consider exploring another market, using another framework, or modifying the topic for another target journal. If an editor has rejected your manuscript because of grammatical problems, consider taking a writing course or consulting with a professional editor. Examine your article and look at the weaknesses the editor indicated. Also, seek peer input from someone who will give it to you honestly.

If your article has been accepted and sent in for publication, consider reslanting your topic for a lay market such as for womens', seniors', and childrens' magazines, or for patient education materials. Nurses have a vast body of knowledge to share, and consumers are interested in what they have to say about health care.

Writing is a skill—anyone can learn it. Remember, you have the information nursing journal editors are seeking . . . and now you have the Process to write it.

EXERCISES

1. Reslant your topic to a lay market and prepare a query letter.
2. Select a topic from your idea file for your next article.

Appendix 1: Selected Publications for Writers

Freelance Writer's Report
CNW Publishing
Maple Ridge Road
North Sandwich, NH 03259

Technical Communication
Journal of the Society for Technical Communication
Suite 304
901 N. Stuart Street
Arlington, VA 22203-1822

The Quill
Journal of the Society of Professional Journalists
P.O. Box 77
Greencastle, IN 46135

The Writer
120 Boylston Street
Boston, MA 02116-4615

Writers Connection
Suite 103
275 Saratoga Avenue
Santa Clara, CA 95050-6664

Writer's Digest
1507 Dana Avenue
Cincinnati, OH 45207

Writer's Journal
27 Empire Drive
St. Paul, MN 55103

Appendix 2: Selected Writing and Literary Associations

American Medical Writers Association (AMWA)
9650 Rockville Pike
Bethesda, MD 20814-3998
(301) 493-0003

American Society of Journalists and Authors, Inc. (ASJA)
1501 Broadway, Suite 302
New York, New York 10036
(212) 997-0947 FAX (212) 768-7414

Association of Biomedical Communication Directors (ABCD)
Penn State University, Educational Resources
P.O. Box 850
Hershey, PA 17033
(717) 531-8345

Association of Medical Illustrators (AMI)
1819 Peachtree Street N.E., Suite 712
Atlanta, GA 30309
(404) 350-7900 FAX (404) 351-3348

California Writers Club
2214 Derby Street
Berkeley, CA 94705

Council of Biology Editors (CBE)
115 LaSalle St., Suite 1400
Chicago, IL 60603-1210
(312) 201-0101 FAX (312) 201-0214

Council for Biomedical Communications Associations
c/o Stewart White, University of Michigan
Biomedical Communications
R 4414, Kresge 0518
Ann Arbor, MI 48109
(313) 763-4686

European Association of Science Editors (EASE)
Box 1897
Lawrence, KS 66044-8897
(913) 843-1235 FAX (913) 843-1274

c/o Maeve O'Connor
49 Rossendale Way
London NW1 OXB, UK
+44(0) 71-388 9668 FAX +44(0) 71-383-3092

Health Sciences Communications Association (HESCA)
6105 Lindell Blvd.
St. Louis, MO 63112
(314) 725-4722

International Association of Business Communicators (IABC)
One Hallidie Plaza, Suite 600
San Francisco, CA 94102
(415) 433-3400 FAX (415) 362-8762

National Association of Science Writers (NASW)
P.O. Box 294
Greenlawn, NY 11740
(516) 757-5664

National Writers Club, Inc. (NWC)
1450 S. Havana, Suite 424
Aurora, CO 80012
(303) 751-7844 FAX (303) 751-8593

Society for Scholarly Publishing (SSP)
10200 W. 44th Ave., Suite 304
Wheat Ridge, CO 80033
(303) 422-3914 FAX (303) 422-8894

Society for Technical Communication (STC)
901 N. Stuart Street, Suite 304
Arlington, VA 22203-1854
(703) 522-4114 FAX (703) 522-2075

Women in Communications, Inc. (WICI)
2101 Wilson Blvd., Suite 417
Arlington, VA 22201
(705) 528-4200 FAX (703) 528-4025

Appendix 3: Health Care Publication Information

The following publication information is compiled from *Business Publication Advertising Source* (1993); *The Cumulative Index to Nursing & Allied Health Literature* (1992); *Literary Market Place* (1994); and *Writer's Market* (1994).

AACN Clinical Issues in Critical Care Nursing
American Association of Critical-Care Nurses
J.B. Lippincott Company
P.O. Box 1600
Hagerstown, MD 21741

AANA Journal
American Association of Nurse Anesthetists
AANA Publishing, Inc.
216 Higgins Road
Park Ridge, IL 60068-5790

AAOHN Journal
American Association of Occupational Health Nurses
Slack, Inc.
6900 Grove Road
Thorofare, NJ 08086-9447

Advance for Nurse Practitioners
Merion Publications, Inc.
650 Park Avenue West
King of Prussia, PA 19406

Advances in Nursing Science
Aspen Publishers, Inc.
7201 McKinney Circle
Frederick, MD 21701

Alternative Health Practitioner: The Journal of
    Complementary and Natural Care
Springer Publishing Company
536 Broadway
New York, NY 10012-3955

American Health Magazine
Reader's Digest Corporation
28 W. 23rd Street
New York, NY 10010

American Journal of Infection Control
Mosby-Year Book, Inc.
11830 Westline Industrial Drive
St. Louis, MO 63146-3318

American Journal of Nursing
American Journal of Nursing Company
555 W. 57th Street
New York, NY 10019-2961

American Journal of Public Health
1015 15th Street, NW
Washington, DC 20005

American Nurse
Suite 100 West
600 Maryland Avenue, SW
Washington, DC 20024-2571

ANNA Journal
American Nephrology Nurses' Association
Box 56
N. Woodbury Road
Pitman, NJ 08071

AORN Journal
Association of Operating Room Nurses, Inc.
10170 E. Mississippi Avenue
Denver, CO 80231

Applied Nursing Research
W.B. Saunders Company
The Curtis Center
Independence Square West
Philadelphia, PA 19106-3399

Archives of Psychiatric Nursing
Yale University School of Nursing
25 Park Street
P.O. Box 9740
New Haven, CT 06536-0740

Aspen's Advisor for Nurse Executives
Aspen Publishers, Inc.
7201 McKinney Circle
Frederick, MD 21701

Better Health
Better Health Press
1450 Chapel Street
New Haven, CT 06511-4440

Bodywise: Magazine of Fitness, Diet, and Preventative Medicine
Prestige Publications, Inc.
4151 Knob Drive
Eagan, MN 55122

Cancer Nursing
University of Florida
College of Nursing
P.O. Box 100187, JHMHC
Gainesville, FL 32610

Cardiovascular Nursing
American Heart Association, Inc.
7320 Greenville Avenue
Dallas, TX 75231

Caring
National Association for Home Care
519 C Street NE
Washington, DC 20002-5809

Case Management Advisor
American Health Consultants, Inc.
3525 Piedmont Road, NE
Building Six, Suite 400
Atlanta, GA 30305

Child & Adolescent Mental Health Care
Springer Publishing Company
536 Broadway
New York, NY 10012-3955

Clinical Nurse Specialist
Williams & Wilkins Company
428 E. Preston Street
Baltimore, MD 21202-3993

Communicating Nursing Research
Western Interstate Commission for Higher Education
P.O. Drawer P
Boulder, CO 80301-9752

Computers in Nursing
J.B. Lippincott Company
P.O. Box 1600
Hagerstown, MD 21741

Contemporary Gerontology
Springer Publishing Company
536 Broadway
New York, NY 10012-3955

Countdown
Juvenile Diabetes Foundation
432 Park Avenue S.
New York, NY 10016

Critical Care Nurse
Cahners Publishing Company
101 Columbia
Aliso Viejo, CA 92656

Critical Care Nursing Clinics of North America
W.B. Saunders Company
The Curtis Center
Independence Square West
Philadelphia, PA 19106-3399

Critical Care Nursing Quarterly
Aspen Publishers, Inc.
7201 McKinney Circle
Frederick, MD 21701

CV Nurse: Trends in Cardiovascular Care
Medical Publishing Enterprises
15-22 Fair Lawn Avenue
Fair Lawn, NJ 07410

DCCN: Dimensions of Critical Care Nursing
Hall Johnson Communications, Inc.
9737 West Ohio Avenue
Lakewood, CO 80226

Death Studies
Dept. of Psychology
Memphis State University
Memphis, TN 38152

Decubitus: The Journal of Skin Ulcers
S-N Publications, Inc.
Communications Building
Second and Main
West Dundee, IL 60118

Dermatology Nursing
Anthony J. Jannetti, Inc.
North Woodbury Road, Box 56
Pitman, NJ 08071

Diabetes Educator
American Association of Diabetes Educators
Suite 1240
444 N. Michigan Avenue
Chicago, IL 60611-3901

Dimensions in Oncology Nursing
Division of Nursing
University of Texas
MD Anderson Cancer Center
1515 Holcombe Boulevard
Houston, TX 77030

Ethics, Law, & Aging
Springer Publishing Company
536 Broadway
New York, NY 10012-3955

FDA Consumer
Food and Drug Administration Publication
5600 Fishers Lane
Rockville, MD 20857

Gastroenterology Nursing
Williams & Wilkins Company
428 E. Preston Street
Baltimore, MD 21202-3993

Geriatric Nursing
American Journal of Care for the Aging
Mosby-Year Book, Inc.
11830 Westline Industrial Drive
St. Louis, MO 63146-3318

Healing Journal
Health Communication Research Institute, Inc.
Suite 105
1050 Fulton Avenue
Sacramento, CA 95825

Health
Time Publishing Ventures
18th Floor
301 Howard Street
San Francisco, CA 94105

Health Care Management Review
Aspen Publishers, Inc.
7201 McKinney Circle
Frederick, MD 21701

Health Care Supervisor
Aspen Publishers, Inc.
7201 McKinney Circle
Frederick, MD 21701

Health Care for Women International
Hemisphere Publishing Corp.
Suite 200
1101 Vermont Avenue
Washington, DC 20005

Health Education Quarterly
John Wiley & Sons, Inc.
605 Third Avenue
New York, NY 10158

Health Progress
Catholic Health Association of U.S.
4455 Woodson Road
St. Louis, MO 63134--3797

Heart and Lung: Journal of Critical Care
Mosby-Year Book, Inc.
11830 Westline Industrial Drive
St. Louis, MO 63146-3318

Holistic Nursing Practice
Aspen Publishers, Inc.
7201 McKinney Circle
Frederick, MD 21701

Home Healthcare Nurse
J.B. Lippincott Company
P.O. Box 1600
Hagerstown, MD 21741

Illness, Crises, and Loss: Multidisciplinary Linkages
Albany Medical Center (A-33)
43 New Scotland Ave.
Albany, NY 12208

Image: Journal of Nursing Scholarship
Sigma Theta Tau International
Honor Society of Nursing, Inc.
550 W. North Street
Indianapolis, IN 46202

Images
American Radiological Nurses Association
Suite 600
2021 Spring Road
Oak Brook, IL 60521

Imprint
National Student Nurses' Association
555 W. 57th Street
New York, NY 10019

Insight
American Society of Ophthalmic Registered Nurses, Inc.
P.O. Box 193030
San Francisco, CA 94119

International Journal of Nursing Studies
Pergamon Press, Inc.
660 White Plains Rd.
Tarrytown, NY 10591-5153

International Nursing Review
3 place Jean-Marteau, CH-1201
Geneva, Switzerland

International Psychogeriatrics
Springer Publishing Company
536 Broadway
New York, NY 10012-3955

Journal of Aging and Ethnicity
Springer Publishing Company
536 Broadway
New York, NY 10012-3955

Journal of the American Academy of Nurse Practitioners
Slack, Inc.
6900 Grove Road
Thorofare, NJ 08086

Journal of the Association of Nurses in AIDS Care
Nursecom, Inc.
1211 Locust Street
Philadelphia, PA 19107

Journal of Burn Care & Rehabilitation
Mosby-Year Book, Inc.
11830 Westline Industrial Drive
St. Louis, MO 63146-3318

Journal of Cancer Education
4125 E. Third Ave.
Denver, CO 80220

Journal of Cardiovascular Nursing
Aspen Publishers, Inc.
7201 McKinney Circle
Frederick, MD 21701

Journal of Case Management
Springer Publishing Company
536 Broadway
New York, NY 10012-3955

Journal of Child and Adolescent Psychiatric and Mental Health Nursing
Nursecom, Inc.
1211 Locust Street
Philadelphia, PA 19107

Journal of Christian Nursing
Nurses Christian Fellowship
P.O. Box 1650
Downers Grove, IL 60515-4634

Journal of Cognitive Psychotherapy
Springer Publishing Company
536 Broadway
New York, NY 10012-3955

Journal of Community Health Nursing
Lawrence Erlbaum Associates, Inc.
365 Broadway
Hillsdale, NJ 07642

Journal of Continuing Education in Nursing
Slack, Inc.
6900 Grove Road
Thorofare, NJ 08086-9447

Journal of Diagnostic Medical Sonography
J.B. Lippincott Company
P.O. Box 1600
Hagerstown, MD 21741

Journal of Emergency Nursing
Mosby-Year Book, Inc.
11830 Westline Industrial Drive
St. Louis, MO 63146-3318

Journal of Ethics, Law, and Aging
Springer Publishing Company
536 Broadway
New York, NY 10012-3955

Journal of Gerontological Nursing
Slack, Inc.
6900 Grove Road
Thorofare, NJ 08086-9447

Journal of Health Economics
Division of Health Policy Research and Education
Harvard University
25 Shattuck St.
Parcel B, 1st Floor
Boston, MA 02115

Journal of Intravenous Nursing
Intravenous Nurses Society
J.B. Lippincott Company
P.O. Box 1600
Hagerstown, MD 21741

Journal of Long Term Home Health Care
Springer Publishing Company
536 Broadway
New York, NY 10012-3955

Journal of Mental Health and Aging
Springer Publishing Company
536 Broadway
New York, NY 10012-3955

Journal of National Black Nurses' Association
P.O. Box 1823
Washington, DC 20001

Journal of Neuroscience Nursing
AANN National Office
Suite 601
224 N. Des Plaines
Chicago, IL 60661

Journal of Nursing Administration
J.B. Lippincott Company
P.O. Box 1600
Hagerstown, MD 21741

Journal of Nursing Care Quality
Aspen Publishers, Inc.
7201 McKinney Circle
Frederick, MD 21701

Journal of Nursing Education
Slack, Inc.
6900 Grove Road
Thorofare, NJ 08086-9447

Journal of Nursing Jocularity
5615 W. Cermak Road
Cicero, IL 60650-2290

Journal of Nursing Measurement
Springer Publishing Company
536 Broadway
New York, NY 10012-3955

Journal of Nursing Staff Development
J.B. Lippincott Company
P.O. Box 1600
Hagerstown, MD 21741

Journal of Nurse-Midwifery
Elsevier Science Publishing Company, Inc.
655 Avenue of the Americas
New York, NY 10010

Journal of Obstetric, Gynecologic, and Neonatal Nursing (JOGNN)
Association of Women's Health, Obstetric and Neonatal Nurses
J.B. Lippincott Company
P.O. Box 1600
Hagerstown, MD 21741

Journal of Ophthalmic Nursing & Technology
Slack, Inc.
6900 Grove Road
Thorofare, NJ 08086-9447

Journal of Pediatric Health Care
National Association of Pediatric Nurses Association and Practitioners
(NAPNAP)
Mosby-Year Book, Inc.
11830 Westline Industrial Drive
St. Louis, MO 63146

Journal of Pediatric Nursing: Nursing Care of Children and Families
W.B. Saunders Company
The Curtis Center
Independence Square West
Philadelphia, PA 19106-3399

Journal of Pediatric Oncology Nursing
W.B. Saunders Company
The Curtis Center
Independence Square West
Philadelphia, PA 19106-3399

Journal of Perinatal and Neonatal Nursing
Aspen Publishers, Inc.
7201 McKinney Circle
Frederick, MD 21701

Journal of Post Anesthesia Nursing
W.B. Saunders Company
The Curtis Center
Independence Square West
Philadelphia, PA 19106-3399

Journal of Practical Nursing
National Association for Practical Nurse Education and Service, Inc.
Suite 310
1400 Spring Street
Silver Spring, MD 20910

Journal of Professional Nursing
American Association of Colleges of Nursing
W.B. Saunders Company
The Curtis Center
Independence Square West
Philadelphia, PA 19106-3399

Journal of Psychosocial Nursing and Mental Health Services
Slack, Inc.
6900 Grove Road
Thorofare, NJ 08086-9447

Journal of School Nursing
Yale University School of Nursing
25 Park Street
P.O. Box 9740
New Haven, CT 06536-0740

Journal of Transcultural Nursing
University of Tennessee
Memphis College of Nursing
877 Madison Avenue
Memphis, TN 38163

Journal of Urological Nursing
International Urological Sciences, Inc.
P.O. Box 408
Long Valley, NJ 07853-0408

Journal of Vascular Nursing
Society for Vascular Nursing, Inc.
Mosby-Year Book, Inc.
11830 Westline Industrial Drive
St. Louis, MO 63146-3318

Journal of Wound, Ostomy, and Continence Nursing
Wound, Ostomy and Continence Nurses Society
Mosby-Year Book, Inc.
11830 Westline Industrial Drive
St. Louis, MO 63146-3318

Longevity
General Media International, Inc.
1965 Broadway
New York, NY 10023-5965

MCN: The American Journal of Maternal Child Nursing
American Journal of Nursing Company
555 W. 57th Street
New York, NY 10019-2961

MEDSURG Nursing
Academy of Medical-Surgical Nurses
Anthony J. Jannetti, Inc.
North Woodbury Road, Box 56
Pitman, NJ 08071

Nurse Anesthetist
Appleton & Lange
P.O. Box 5630
Norwalk, CT 06856

Nurse Author & Editor
Hall Johnson Communications, Inc.
9737 W. Ohio Avenue
Lakewood, CO 80226

Nurse Educator
J.B. Lippincott Company
P.O. Box 1600
Hagerstown, MD 21741

Nurse Practitioner: American Journal of Primary Health Care
Elsevier Science Publishing Company, Inc.
6555 Avenue of the Americas
New York, NY 10010

Nurse Practitioner Forum
W.B. Saunders Company
The Curtis Center
Independence Square West
Philadelphia, PA 19106-3399

Nurses' Drug Alert
M.J. Powers & Company
374 Millburn Avenue
Millburn, NJ 07041-1343

NurseWeek/California Nursing Review
1156-C Aster Avenue
Sunnyvale, CA 94086

Nursing
Springhouse Corp.
111 Bethlehem Pike, P.O. Box 908
Springhouse, PA 19477-0908

Nursing (London): The Journal of Clinical Practice,
  Education and Management
Mark Allen Publishing Ltd.,
Croxted Mews
288 Croxted Road
London SE24 9DA
England

Nursing '95 (Title appears with year, e.g. Nursing '94)
Springhouse Corporation
P.O. Box 908
1111 Bethlehem Pike
Springhouse, PA 19477-0908

Nursing Administration Quarterly
Aspen Publishers, Inc,
7201 McKinney Circle
Frederick, MD 21701

Nursing Clinics of North America
W.B. Saunders Company
The Curtis Center
Independence Square West
Philadelphia, PA 19106-3399

Nursing Diagnosis
J.B. Lippincott Company
P.O. Box 1600
Hagerstown, MD 21741

Nursing Economic$
Anthony J. Jannetti, Inc.
North Woodbury Road, Box 56
Pitman, NJ 08071

Nursing Educators Microworld
13740 Harleigh Court
Saratoga, CA 95070

Nursing Forum
Nursecom, Inc.
1211 Locust Street
Philadelphia, PA 19107

Nursing and Health Care
National League for Nursing
350 Hudson Street
New York, NY 10014

Nursing Leadership Forum
Springer Publishing Company
536 Broadway
New York, NY 10012-3955

Nursing Management
S-N Publications, Inc.
Suite 200
103 N. Second Street
Dundee, IL 60118-2002

Nursing Outlook
Mosby-Year Book, Inc.
11830 Westline Industrial Drive
St. Louis, MO 63146-3318

Nursing Quality Connection
Mosby-Year Book, Inc.
11830 Westline Industrial Drive
St. Louis, MO 63146-3318

Nursing Research
American Journal of Nursing Company
P.O. Box 1728
Riverton, NJ 08077-7328

Nursing Science Quarterly
Chestnut House Publications
P.O. Box 22492
Pittsburg, PA 15222-0492

Nursing Times
Macmillan Magazines
4 Little Essex Street
London WC2R 3LF
England

Nursingworld Journal
Prime National Publishing corporation
470 Boston Post Road
Weston, MA 02193

Oncology Nursing Forum
Oncology Nursing Society
Oncology Nursing Press, Inc.
501 Holiday Drive
Pittsburg, PA 15220-2749

Online Journal of Knowledge Synthesis for Nursing
3434 W. Penn St.
Philadelphia, PA 19129
e-mail:barnsthr@son.nursing.uppen.edu

OR Manager
P.O. Box 17487
Boulder, CO 80308-7487

Orthopaedic Nursing
Anthony J. Jannetti, Inc.
North Woodbury Road, Box 56
Pitman, NJ 08071

Ostomy/Wound Management
Health Management Publications, Inc.
550 American Avenue
King of Prussia, PA 19406

Pediatric Nursing
Anthony J. Jannetti, Inc.
North Woodbury Road, Box 56
Pitman, NJ 08071

Perspectives in Psychiatric Care
Nursecom, Inc.
1211 Locust Street
Philadelphia, PA 19106

Plastic Surgical Nursing
Anthony J. Jannetti, Inc.
North Woodbury Road, Box 56
Pitman, NJ 08071

Progress in Cardiovascular Nursing
International Publishing Group
P.O. Box 3000, Dept. PC
Denville, NJ 07834

Public Health Nursing
Blackwell Scientific Publications, Ltd.
Suite 208
3 Cambridge Center
Cambridge, MA 02142

Recruitment & Retention Report
Hall Johnson Communications, Inc.
9737 W. Ohio Avenue
Lakewood, CO 80226

Reflections
Sigma Theta Tau International
Honor Society of Nursing
550 W. North Street
Indianapolis, IN 46202

Rehabilitation Nursing Research
Association of Rehabilitation Nurses
First Floor
5700 Old Orchard Road
Skokie, IL 60077-1057

Rehabilitation Psychology
Springer Publishing Company
536 Broadway
New York, NY 10012-3955

Rescue
Jems Communications
P.O. Box 2789
Carlsbad, CA 92018-2789

Research in Nursing & Health
John Wiley & Sons, Inc.
605 Third Avenue
New York, NY 10158

RN
Medical Economics Publishing
P.O. Box 2119
Marion, OH 43305-2119

Rogerian Nursing Science News
Society of Rogerian Scholars, Inc.
P.O. Box 362
Prince Street Station
New York, NY 10012-0007

School Nurse
Health Information Publications, Inc.
92 S. Highland Avenue
Ossining, NY 10562

Scholarly Inquiry for Nursing Practice
Springer Publishing Company, Inc.
536 Broadway
New York, NY 10012-3955

SCI Nursing
American Association of Spinal Cord Injury Nurses
75-20 Astoria Boulevard
Jackson Heights, NY 11370-1177

Seminars in Oncology Nursing
W.B. Saunders Company
The Curtis Center
Independence Square West
Philadelphia, PA 19106-3399

Seminars in Perioperative Nursing
W.B. Saunders Company
The Curtis Center
Independence Square West
Philadelphia, PA 19106-3399

Shape Magazine
Weider Health & Fitness
21100 Erwin Street
Woodland Hills, CA 91367

Staff Development Insider
Mosby-Year Book, Inc.
11830 Westline Industrial Drive
St. Louis, MO 63146-3318

Thanatos
Association of Death Education & Counseling
P.O. Box 6009
Tallahassee, FL 32314

The Nurse, The Patient, & The Law
Cox Publications
P.O. Box 20316
Billings, MT 59104-0316

Today's OR Nurse
Slack, Inc.
6900 Grove Road
Thorofare, NJ 08086-9447

Urologic Nursing
Mosby-Year Book, Inc.
11830 Westline Industrial Drive
St. Louis, MO 63146-3318

Vim & Vigor: America's Family Health Magazine
Suite 11
8805 N. 23rd Avenue
Phoenix, AZ 85021

Weight Watcher's Magazine
11th Floor
360 Lexington Avenue
New York, NY 10017

Western Journal of Nursing Research
Sage Publications, Inc.
2455 Teller Road
Newbury Park, CA 91320

Your Health
Globe Communications Corp.
5401 NW Broken Sound Boulevard
Boca Raton, FL 33487

Your Health
Meridian International, Inc.
Box 10010
Ogden, UT 84409

Your Health & Fitness
General Learning Corp.
60 Revere Drive
Northbrook, IL 60062-1563

Index

Ⓢ *Springer Publishing Company*

A Nurse's Guide to Public Speaking
Barry Kaplan, MFA

This information-packed concise guide, designed especially for nurses, can help you prepare to be a confident and effective public speaker. It outlines concrete steps you can take to prepare for and deliver a speech or lecture. Hon-est and illuminating quotes from prominent nurses on their experiences as speakers are given throughout the book.

Contents: What to Know Before You Make Your Speech • Prepare Your Speech • Prepare Yourself • Breaking the Fear Barrier • Making the Speech • Who Owns the Speech • Transforming a Speech into a Paper, a Paper into a Speech • Other Forms of Oral Communication

1997   120pp (est.)   0-8261-9590-3   *softcover*

Successful Grant Writing
Strategies for Health and Human Service Professionals
Laura N. Gitlin, PhD and **Kevin J. Lyons,** PhD

This book guides the reader through the language and basic components of grantmanship. It illustrates how to develop ideas for funding, write the sections of a proposal, organize different types of project structures, and finally, how to understand the review process. Each chapter describes a specific aspect of grantmanship and suggests innovative strategies to implement the information that is presented. The appendices contain helpful materials, such as a list of key acronyms, examples of timelines and sample budget sheets. The strategies in this volume are beneficial to individuals and departments in academic, clinical, or community-based settings.

Partial Contents: Becoming Familiar with Funding Sources • Developing Your Ideas for Funding • Learning about Your Institution • Common Sections of Proposals • Preparing a Budget • Technical Considerations • Strategies for Effective Writing • Understanding the Process of Collaboration • Understanding the Review Process

1996   235pp   0-8261-9260-2   *hard cover*

536 Broadway, New York, NY 10012-3955 • (212) 431-4370 • Fax (212) 941-7842

Springer Publishing Company

The Nurse Consultant's Handbook
Belinda Puetz, PhD, RN
Linda J. Shinn, MBA, RN, CAE

What is a consultant? What type of person makes a successful consultant? How does one launch and manage one's own business as a consultant? This manual answers these questions and provides comprehensive guidelines and practical information on becoming a nurse consultant.

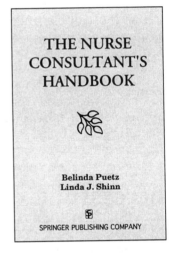

The authors, both experienced consultants, outline the consultation process in detail, describe the business and financial savvy required, and give tips on marketing and pricing one's services, making presentations, networking, and managing one's personal life in relation to one's career. The book addresses independent entrepreneurs as well as "intrapreneurs" who consult as an inside member of a larger organization.

Contents:
- What is Consultation?
- The Consultation Process
- Preparation for Consultation: Planning a Career Path
- The Internal Nurse Consultant
- Starting a Consulting Business
- Marketing Consultation Services
- Networking
- Legal and Ethical Aspects of Consulting
- The Consultant as a Person

1997   248pp   0-8261-9520-2   Hard

536 Broadway, New York, NY 10012-3955 • (212) 431-4370 • Fax (212) 941-7842